T0320671

Hand Hygiene Practices in Schools

This book provides essential guidance to help schools in developing countries to promote and maintain hand hygiene practices, thus reducing the prevalence of infectious diseases such as diarrhoea and respiratory infection that cause both illness and absenteeism.

Discussing both the challenges that hinder hand hygiene practices and the opportunities available to promote positive behaviours, it is particularly timely since the onset of the global COVID-19 pandemic, where infection could also be passed on through the hands. Drawing on both evidence-based research and successful interventions in specific countries, the book builds to offer a best-practice manual to address this important issue.

This will be ideal reading for public health and community health workers in developing regions, as well as those working for NGOs.

Balwani Chingatichifwe Mbakaya is an Associate Professor in the Department of Public Health, Faculty of Applied Sciences, University of Livingstonia in Malawi. He is also a Senior Adjunct Lecturer in the Faculty of Health Sciences at Mzuzu University, Malawi. Professor Balwani is a public health specialist with a bias in field epidemiology and has held different academic and administrative positions in government and health-related training institutions such as in Christian Health Association of Malawi (CHAM) (St John's Institute for Health, Holly Family College of Nursing, and Ekwendeni College of Health Sciences). The author has also taught as an adjunct lecturer at St John of God College, Mulanje Mission College and Nkhoma Mission College. The author has written extensively and published high-profile research in reputable journals such as *PLOS ONE, BMC, BMJ, IJERPH,* and *AJIC.*

Hand Hygiene Practices in Schools

A Guide to Best-Practice in
Developing Countries

Balwani Chingatichifwe Mbakaya

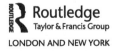

Routledge
Taylor & Francis Group

LONDON AND NEW YORK

First published 2023
by Routledge
4 Park Square, Milton Park, Abingdon, Oxon OX14 4RN

and by Routledge
605 Third Avenue, New York, NY 10158

Routledge is an imprint of the Taylor & Francis Group, an informa business

British Library Cataloguing-in-Publication Data
A catalogue record for this book is available from the British Library

ISBN: 978-1-032-34229-0 (hbk)
ISBN: 978-1-032-45085-8 (pbk)
ISBN: 978-1-003-37531-9 (ebk)

DOI: 10.4324/b23319

Typeset in Bembo
by codeMantra

This book is dedicated to my late father (Binalawo Nkhonjera) and late mother (Lyness Mhango) for their kindness, love, care, encouragement, guidance and support for me to reach this far in life. Your grandchildren (Viwemi, Temwanani & Temweka), daughter in-law (Temwani Luhanga) and I miss you very much dear parents. May your souls continue resting in eternal peace till we meet again.

Contents

Figures

Tables

Contributors

Master R.O. Chisale is a Senior Lecturer in the field of Microbiology and Immunology in the Faculty of Science Technology and Innovations under Biological Sciences department at Mzuzu University. Through the research, he primarily strives to address health disparities among underserved communities where quality health is highly sorted after. His research work involves collaborative partnerships with national, regional and international institutions and working with both private and public institutions. His teaching areas include microbiology (general and medical), immunology, public health, epidemiology, research bioethics as well as laboratory quality management systems. Master Chisale has BSc in Biomedical Sciences, MSc in Medicine Majoring Microbiology and has published over 20 research work in highly reputable peer-reviewed journals.

Sheena Ramazanu is a Research Fellow at the Alice Lee Centre for Nursing Studies, Yong Loo Lin School of Medicine, National University of Singapore. Through her research, Dr Sheena strives to optimise health capacities of underserved communities. Her research studies involve collaborative partnerships with national, regional and international institutions. Dr Sheena's teaching areas focus on health promotion, professional nursing ethics and law, and honours degree thesis supervision. She pursued her nursing degree from the Singapore Institute of Technology, University of Manchester and attained a first-class honour. She was presented with an Outstanding Dissertation Achievement Award. From 2014 to 2016, Sheena received University of Manchester Full Scholarship to pursue Master's in Clinical Research. Sheena was awarded the prestigious and competitive Hong Kong PhD fellowship from 2017 to 2020. Dr Sheena received several awards, including the Ministry of Health Gold Medal Award, Tay Eng Soon Health Sciences Award, WorldSkills Singapore Silver Medal in Caring, Singapore Nurses Association Award, and Capital Land Healthcare Frontlines Award.

Foreword

The author of this book consolidates existing evidence from best practice in the field of hand hygiene. Observing the challenges that hand hygiene practice faces especially in school settings in developing countries, efforts are made by the author of this book to unveil the challenges and offer solutions based on best practice from studies conducted worldwide. He further describes the possible recommended strategies for utilisation. Lessons from developed countries where adoption of hand hygiene is doing well are incorporated into this book.

The motivation to write this book emanated from the author's doctoral study. During his doctoral candidature, the author did his practicum in special school in Hong Kong, promoting hand hygiene in order to prevent infection and school absenteeism among children with mild intellectual disability. The author also promoted weight management among the same group of students under the health promoting school concept. The author further implemented a school-based hand hygiene programme (HHP) in Malawi, sub-Saharan Africa using a randomised controlled trial with an embedded qualitative design. Thus, the author has in-depth knowledge and expertise in implementing hand hygiene programmes.

Preface

Over the past decade, hand hygiene has been touted to be at the centre of infection prevention. This has also been recently emphasised by World Health Organization (WHO) as a way of preventing diarrhoea and respiratory conditions among schoolchildren. Consequently, reducing school absenteeism which comes due to these infections hence improves school attendance and performance. The significance of hand hygiene has been vindicated by the emerging and re-emerging several of respiratory infections such as COVID-19 and influenza, just to mention but a few.

This book is about scientific basis and practice to promote hand hygiene in schools, and offer guidance to best practice in developing countries. Anyone involved in promoting hand hygiene among schoolchildren in developing countries can use this book. Trainees in health profession can benefit from this book too. Academicians can use this book as a reference when delivering their lessons to health trainees.

This book contains the following;

- An overview of hand hygiene
- The encyclopaedia of hand hygiene
- Status of hand hygiene practices among schoolchildren in developing countries
- Factors influencing hand hygiene practices among schoolchildren in developing countries
- Opportunities to embrace hand hygiene practices among schoolchildren
- Lessons derived from developed countries
- Recommended strategies to improve hand hygiene compliance among schoolchildren in developing countries
- Way forward

Acknowledgements

First, I would like to thank my wife Temwani, our first born Viwemi, and our second born twins Temwanani and Temweka, for your endurance during the time I focussed on writing this book. You gave me space each time I wanted to concentrate on writing. You socially, psychologically and economically supported me during this long journey of writing this book. I do not take your support for granted and I owe you a lot.

Second, I would like to sincerely thank Professor Regina Lee and Dr Paul Lee for motivating and encouraging me to focus my career in the field of hand hygiene among schoolchildren. Your supervision during my PhD studies led to the conception of the idea that finally has materialised into a book.

Lastly, I would like to thank parents, schoolchildren, teachers and school authorities in Malawi who allowed me to interact with the schoolchildren and share the experiences in this book.

Abbreviations

CDC	Centers for Disease Control and Prevention
CHAM	Christian Health Association of Malawi Children's Emergency Fund
COVID-19	Coronavirus Disease 2019
HHP	Hand Hygiene Programme
ISAMA	Independent School Association of Malawi
SBHHP	School-Based Hand Hygiene Programme
UNESCO	United Nations Educational, Scientific and Cultural Organization
UNICEF	United Nations Children's Fund (formerly; United Nations International)
WASH	Water, Sanitation and Hygiene
WHO	World Health Organization

1   Overview of hand hygiene

The value of hand hygiene

Hand hygiene can minimise the number of microorganisms on the hands surface, in return reducing the incidence of diarrhoea, respiratory infection and consequently school absenteeism (Luby et al., 2004; Luby et al., 2005; Patel et al., 2012; Zhang, Mosa, Hayward, & Mathews, 2013). This means that if correct hand hygiene interventions can be scaled up globally, especially in school settings in developing countries, the lives of many children could be saved, and morbidity reduced.

Hand hygiene has been identified and acknowledged as the most effective intervention to lower the transmission of pathogens in school community (Morton & Schultz, 2004; World Health Organization [WHO], 2009; Lee & Lee, 2014). However, poor hand hygiene compliance has been observed in young children; most children fail to perceive the importance of hand washing to their health and wellness (Lopez-Quintero, Freeman, & Neumark, 2009).

According to the Centers for Disease Control and Prevention [CDC], the Center for Health and Health Care in Schools [CHHCS] (2007), hand washing is the single most effective practice a person can adopt to reduce the spread of infectious diseases and they further report that failure to sufficiently wash hands contributes to nearly 50% of all food-borne illness outbreaks. A study led by Borchgrevink, Cha, and Kim (2013) reported that only 5% of people washed their hands enough to kill infectious pathogens and illness-causing germs after using the toilets, as most people splash-and-go when it comes to hand washing. The same study also found that 33% of hand washers did not use soap and 10% skipped hand washing altogether.

Several studies have found that a hand washing program is a community alleviation measure that can reduce influenza illness in the event of a severe pandemic (Kampf & Kramer, 2004; Lee et al., 2010). With the current COVID-19 pandemic, hand washing becomes one of the major recommendations to curb the spread of the disease (WHO, 2020). Proper hand washing technique is effective in preventing the transmission of communicable diseases (Rabie & Curtis, 2006).

DOI: 10.4324/b23319-1

The development of a structural hand washing protocol as a key component of a hand hygiene program was associated with reduced school community outbreak rates (Center for Health Protection, 2007), including respiratory tract infections and pandemic influenza A/H1N1 virus in years 2006, 2008, and 2009. Infectious agents contracted by schoolchildren reportedly led to infections in up to 50% of household members (Aiello, Larson, & Sedlak, 2008). This means that if much effort can be made to promote hand hygiene among schoolchildren, the approach can help reduce morbidity not only among schoolchildren but also the community at large, because schoolchildren could be the source of transmission of infections from school settings to their household.

A structural hand washing program is a community alleviation measure to reduce influenza illness, as well as COVID-19 in the event of a severe pandemic, because children in school settings are 18 times more likely to contract pathogens than those who stay at home (Bylinsky, 1994).

Hand hygiene is a key component of good hygiene practice at household level, school settings and the community at large, and can produce significant benefits in terms of reducing the incidence of infection, most particularly gastrointestinal infections but also respiratory tract and skin infections (Bloomfield, Aiello, Cookson, O'Boyle, & Larson, 2007).

Addressing challenges that affect hand hygiene among schoolchildren is vital in promoting health and reducing school absenteeism caused by infectious diseases such as diarrhoea and respiratory conditions. The information contained in this book will help to inform school health workers, education system, policy makers, and governments enabling them to categorise and prioritise activities into viable strategies when implementing hand hygiene interventions in school settings. The information in this book will also be useful to researchers, academicians and trainees in the health field.

Why this book?

This book guides public health workers, community health workers, environmental health officers, health and safety personnel, and teachers working within school settings in resource-deprived areas. The information here in contained will help the named group of service providers in promoting hand hygiene practices among schoolchildren in school settings in order to reduce the prevalence of infectious diseases such as diarrhoea and respiratory conditions, which are transmissible through contaminated hands. The information here in contained is based on best practice and evidence from reliable literature. The book emphasises on the importance of hand hygiene practices in prevention of infectious diseases such as diarrhoea and respiratory infection in school settings. Challenges that hinder hand hygiene practices as well as opportunities available to promote hand hygiene behaviours are also discussed.

Developing countries especially in sub-Saharan Africa have the highest prevalence of infectious diseases such as diarrhoea and respiratory infections, which claims more death in children in the world. Hence, this book becomes more relevant for application in developing countries where the burden of infectious diseases is huge; yet hand hygiene is simple and the most cost-effective intervention to reduce the burden of both diarrhoea and respiratory conditions, and in return reduce school absenteeism among children. Hand washing with soap can reduce the risk of diarrhoea by 42%–48% (Cairncross et al., 2010).

Effective and appropriate hand hygiene practice for schoolchildren is important in preventing infectious diseases such as diarrhoea, which is the second most common cause of death among school-age children in sub-Saharan Africa (Rao, Lopez, & Hemed, 2006). Because lifestyle and behavioural choices are shaped in childhood, it is important that health education about hand hygiene be introduced very early to influence healthy behaviours (Lee, Loke, Wu, & Ho, 2010). This is possible to achieve in children because their poor hygiene habits are less established, unlike adults, whose habits are firmly grounded and difficult or unlikely to change (Eshuchi, 2013). Hence, the focus of this book is primarily targeted at young children in school settings.

Well-practiced and consistent hand washing techniques can produce significant benefits in reducing incidence of gastrointestinal and respiratory infections (Bloomfield et al., 2007). In turn, this can lead to reductions in morbidity and mortality rates, as well as in school absenteeism among children (Cairncross et al., 2010). Consequently, this may lead to an improvement in their school performance, which may in the end have positive implications for development in their countries (Malawi Demographic & Health Survey (MDHS), 2002). Studies have revealed that students who are absent frequently or for long periods are likely to have difficulty mastering the material presented in class, making absenteeism an important education issue (MDHS, 2002). Therefore, hand washing has the simultaneous benefit of improving both education and health (WHO, 2009).

It is important therefore that this book serves as a guide to education, policy and practice in order to help in promoting hand hygiene uptake among schoolchildren and the general community.

References

Borchgrevink, C.P., Cha, J., & Kim, S. (2013). Hand washing practices in a college town environment. *J. Environ. Health* **2013**, Apr;*75*(8), 18–24. PMID: 23621052.

Bloomfield, S.F., Aiello, A.E., Cookson, B., O'Boyle, C., & Larson, E.L. (2007). The effectiveness of hand hygiene procedures in reducing the risk of infections in homes and community settings including handwashing and alcohol-based hand sanitizers. *Am. J. Infect. Control* **2007**, *35*, S27–S64.

Bylinsky, G. (1994). The new fight against killer microbes. *Fortune* 1994, *130*(5), 74–82

Cairncross, S., Hunt, C., Boisson, S., Bostoen, K., Curtis, V., Fung, I.C., & Schmidt, W.-P. (2010). Water, sanitation and hygiene for the prevention of diarrhea. *Int. J. Epidemiol.* 2010, *39*, i193–i205.

Centre for Health Protection (2007). Proper hand hygiene. Retrieved from http://www.chp.gov.hk/en/content/9/460/19728.html.

Curtis, V., Cairncross, S. (2003). Effect of washing hands with soap on diarrhoea risk in the community: A systematic review. *Lancet Infect Dis.* 2003, *3*(5), 275-81.

Eshuchi, R.C.E. (2013). Promoting handwashing with soap behaviour in Kenyan Schools: Learning from puppetry trials among primary school children in Kenya. Available online: http://eprints.qut.edu.au/62022/1/Rufus_Eshuchi_Thesis.pdf (accessed on 15 December 2015).

Kampf, G., & Kramer, A. (2004). Epidemiologic background of hand hygiene and evaluation of the most important agents for scrubs and rubs. *Clin. Microbiol. Rev.* 2004, Oct;17(4), 863–893, table of contents. doi:10.1128/CMR.17.4.863–893.2004. PMID: 15489352; PMCID: PMC523567.

Lee, R.L.T., & Lee, P.H. (2014). To evaluate the effects of a simplified hand washing improvement program in schoolchildren with mild intellectual disability: A pilot study. *Res. Dev. Disbil.* 2014, doi:10/1016/j.ridd.2014.07.016.

Lee, R.L., Loke, A.Y., Wu, C.S., & Ho, A.P. (2010). The lifestyle behaviours and psychosocial well-being of primary school students in Hong Kong. *J. Clin. Nurs.* 2010, *19*, 1462–1472.

Lopez-Quintero C., Freeman P., & Neumark Y. (2009). Hand washing among school children in Bogotá, Colombia. *Am. J. Public Health* 2009, Jan; *99*(1), 94-101. doi: 10.2105/AJPH.2007.129759.

Luby, S.P., Agboatwalla, M., Feikin, D.R., Painter, J., Billhimer, W., Altaf, A., & Hoekstra, R.M. (2005). Effect of hand washing on children's health: A randomised controlled trial. *The Lancet* 2005, *366*, 225–233.

Luby, S.P., Agboatwalla, M., Painter, J., Altaf, A., Billhimer, W.L., & Hoekstra, R.M. (2004). Effect of intensive handwashing promotion on childhood diarrhea in high-risk communities in Pakistan: A randomized controlled trial. *JAMA* 2004, *291*, 2547–2554.

Malawi Demographic & Health Survey: Education Data for Decision Making. (2002). Available online: http://pdf.usaid.gov/pdf_docs/pnacr009.pdf (accessed on 15 February 2016).

Morton, J.L., & Schultz, A.A. (2004). Healthy hands: Use of an alcohol gel as an adjunct to handwashing in elementary school children. *J. Sch. Nurs.* 2004, *20*, 161–167.

Patel, M.K., Harris, J.R., Juliao, P., Nygren, B., Were, V., Kola, S., & Quick, R. (2012). Impact of a hygiene curriculum and the installation of simple handwashing and drinking water stations in rural Kenyan primary schools on student health and hygiene practices. *Am. J. Trop. Med. Hyg.* 2012, *87*, 594–601.

Rabie, T., & Curtis, V. (2006). Handwashing and risk of respiratory infections: A quantitative systematic review. *Trop. Med. Int. Health* 2006, *11*, 258–267.

Rao, C., Lopez, A.D., & Hemed, Y. (2006). Causes of death. In *Disease and Mortality in Sub-Saharan Africa*, 2nd ed.; Jamison, D.T., Feachem, R.G., Makgoba, M.W., Bos, E.R., Baingana, F.K., Hofman, K.J., & Rogo, K.O., Eds; The

International Bank for Reconstruction and Development/The World Bank: Washington, DC, USA, 2006; Chapter 5.

The Center for Health and Health Care in Schools [CHHCS] (2007). Advancing School-Connected Strategies for Children's Health and School Success. https://healthinschools.org/

WHO. (2009). A guide to the implementation of the WHO multimodal hand hygiene improvement strategy, 2009. Available online: http://www.who.int/gpsc/5may/Guide_to_Implementation.pdf (accessed on 19 December 2015).

WHO. (2020). Hand washing an effective tool to prevent COVID-19, other diseases. Accessed from https://www.who.int/southeastasia/news/detail/15-10-2020-handwashing-an-effective-tool-to-prevent-covid-19-other-diseases

Zhang, C., Mosa, A.J., Hayward, A.S., & Mathews, S.A. (2013). Promoting clean hands among children in Uganda: A school-based intervention using "tippy-taps". *Public Health* **2013**, *127*, 586–589.

2 The encyclopaedia of hand hygiene – what it is all about?

Definition of hand hygiene

Hand hygiene is a general term applied to the use of soap or solution, which can be non-antimicrobial or have an antimicrobial effect, and water, or a waterless antimicrobial agent, to the surface of the hands. On the other hand, hand washing is defined as washing hands with plain or antimicrobial soap and water (World Health Organization [WHO], 2009). Hand hygiene is the act of keeping our hands clean and free from microorganisms. The process is achieved through the use of clean water and soap or hand rub using hand sanitisers, which reduce contamination on hands by removal or killing the organisms in situ.

Hand hygiene can therefore be grouped into two main types. First, the use of hand washing, which can be done with antibacterial soap (recommended) or plain soap. The soap can be in the form of liquid, which is recommended, or tablet which is prone to contamination because everyone touches it at each episode of washing hands. Some resource constraint communities have gone to the extent of using ash or sand/mud and water in trying to keep their hand clean and free from microorganisms. The efficacy/effectiveness is yet to be proved of such practices. Rigorous research studies such as ran-domised controlled trials (RCTs) need to be carried out in this area to ascertain the efficacy of using ash or sand/mud for hand washing. Second, a hand rub using hand sanitisers has proven to be effective in keeping the hands free from microorganisms. Hand sanitisers can be alcohol based or non-alcohol based which are preferred in Muslim communities.

Comparison between hand rub and hand washing with soap

One of the studies (Pickering, et al., 2013), in which a comparison was made between waterless hand sanitiser and hand washing with water and soap, found that students at schools with sanitisers were 23% less likely to have observed diarrhoea than control students (p = 0.02). Pickering et al. (2013) further found that hand sanitiser was significantly better than hand washing with respect to reductions in levels of fecal streptococci

DOI: 10.4324/b23319-2

Table 2.1 Comparison between the utilisation of hand washing and hand sanitiser

Hand washing	Hand sanitiser
Used in both visibly dirty hands or not	Convenient where hands are not visibly dirty
Relatively cheaper	Relatively expensive
A procedure/technique is needed	Relatively easy to use
A must in school settings in developing countries	Not ideal in school settings in developing countries with resource constraint and poor environment
Used in all settings where hand washing facilities are available	Convenient in hospital settings
Cultural universality	Sanitisers with alcohol content faces cultural resistance especially in Muslim communities

Source: Assoc. Prof. Mbakaya

(p=0.01). The use of hand sanitiser is also regarded as user friendly in hospital settings (Golin, Choi, & Ghahary, 2020). In developing countries, it could be a challenge sometimes to acquire a hand sanitiser which is relatively expensive compared to the use of soap and water.

But hand washing is recommended in situations where hands are visibly dirty. This is the case in most developing countries where schools in rural areas do not have enough facilities including poor surroundings. As such, hand washing with soap and water could be the best option (Table 2.1).

Despite the differences outlined as above, both hand washing and hand sanitiser share a common goal, that is, to keep the hands clean and break the chain of infectious disease transmission. Such diseases include diarrhoea and respiratory infections. However, hand washing with water and soap is recommended in school settings of developing countries. This is because the school environment is generally poor due to limited resources. As such, schoolchildren's hands are visibly dirty most of the time, which cannot be kept clean merely by using hand sanitiser.

Sources of water and hand hygiene facilities in school settings

School settings in developing countries have varied settings for hand washing, ranging from temporary to permanent. Some of the examples of such settings are a sink with running water from taps, tippy-taps and buckets. Therefore, the section that follows describes the settings listed above.

- *Tap water*: It is a very clean source because it washes to drain, but its use varies by the type of soap used, that is liquid versus tablet. The only challenge with tap water is that the coverage is very low in developing countries, especially in rural settings where the majority of school-aged children reside. Most schools in developing countries do not have running water or may have dry taps. However, in situations where clean water from a tap is available, usually the challenge becomes the availability of soap. A hand washing station with tap water from a clean source is the best setting and should be advocated for. See Figure 2.1 of a locally constructed sink using available and accessible resources such as sand, locally made bricks and cement. It is therefore recommended that school authority, teachers and parents through committees such as Parent Teacher Association (PTA) should prioritise resource mobilisation to make sure that schools have such basic structure for children to use when washing hands.

- *Tippy-taps*: The first tippy-tap was constructed by Dr Jim Watt and Jackson Masawi of the Salvation Army in Chiweshe, Zimbabwe, and was termed the Mukombe in the 1980s. The Mukombe is a type of gourd or calabash, which is used as a can (Morgan, 2013). Tippy-taps

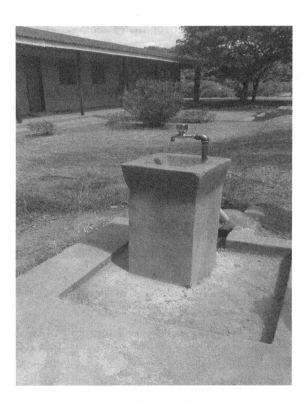

Figure 2.1 An example of a simple hand washing station with clean running water constructed outside the classroom in Northern Malawi.
Source: Assoc. Prof. Mbakaya.

are simple and economic hand washing stations made with locally available materials such as plastic containers, jerry cans and gourds, and do not depend on a piped water supply (Eshuchi, 2013). Biran (2011) describes a tippy-tap as

> *a device consisting of a small (three or five-litre) jerry can be filled with water and suspended from a wooden frame. A string is attached to the neck of the jerry can that can be tied to a piece of wood at ground level. Pressing on this piece of wood with the foot, tips the jerry can to release a stream of water through a small hole. Soap is suspended from the frame beside the jerry can*

• Some of the advantages of tippy-taps are as follows: it is easy to construct, it utilises very little water; it is easier to use and only soap is touched, thereby making hand washing very hygienic because it avoids contamination of the jerry can, unlike the real tap (Biran, 2011) (see Figure 2.2.).

Tippy-taps could be a technology of choice for promoting hand hygiene through hand washing in school settings in developing countries. This practice would consequently reduce diarrhoea and respiratory disorders and deaths that are associated with the lack of water, inadequate hand washing stations and limited resources (Pickering et al., 2013).

Tippy-taps, although simply constructed from locally affordable and accessible materials, could be the suitable hand washing stations for school settings in resource-constrained regions that often lack adequate water for hand washing. The average amount of water used for hand washing using

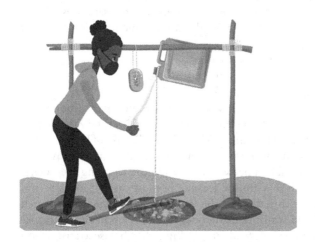

Figure 2.2 An example of a tippy-tap.
Source: UNICEF South Africa, Children's Radio Foundation. (June, 2020).

tippy-taps is far much less compared to ordinary hand washing stations such as taps. Comparatively, a good hand wash using tippy-tap may use only 50 ml of water, while washing hands using tap water may utilise up to 500 ml of water (Morgan, 2013). Furthermore, tippy-taps could help in increasing hand washing behaviour in schools because it is appealing, humorous and easy to use for children, in turn reducing the number of deaths in children that occur due to poor health conditions associated with hand hygiene practices (Biran, 2011). In addition, tippy-tap may reduce school absenteeism that come in because of illnesses that affect school-children, in turn improving school attendance and child performance as well as contributing positively to the development of their respective countries. Enabling technology is one of the factors that externally influence individual's probability to accomplish a behaviour (Biran, 2011). The UNICEF and WaterAid recommended the use of tippy-taps in schools and family houses next to the latrines (UNICEF, 2011; WaterAid, 2012). Tippy-taps are possibly the best known low-cost enabling technology for hand washing (Biran, 2011) and currently, these are commonly used in Eastern and Southern African countries like Uganda, Rwanda and Zambia (WaterAid, 2012).

Tippy-tap is clean and hygienic because it washes to drain but depends on the source of water. Tippy-tap is also cheap and can be a good alternative to hand wash basins in settings where resources are difficult to locate.

Below is a summary of some of the advantages of tippy-taps (UNICEF, 2020)

1   Provide running water and soap for hand washing
2   Provide water drainage
3   Have a hands-free tap
4   Can be easily reached by children and people with disabilities
5   Can be built 2 metres apart to keep physical distancing for COVID-19 prevention
6   Are cost effective and durable in a crisis
7   Are easy to move, put together and taken apart
8   Don't need specialised building skills.
   • *Buckets*: The use of a bucket with a tap is becoming common nowadays, especially with the coming in of the COVID-19 pandemic. With good care and clean source of water, the use of buckets with a tap can serve the purpose of promoting hand hygiene. However, cleanliness is doubtful because it may require cleaning the bucket everyday which may not be feasible in most cases. This may end up in the contamination of the water stored in buckets. In such scenarios, hand washing using buckets could aid in the transmission of infections, instead of breaking the disease transmission cycle. In addition, use of a bucket may depend on the source of water despite cleaning the bucket. For example, using water from

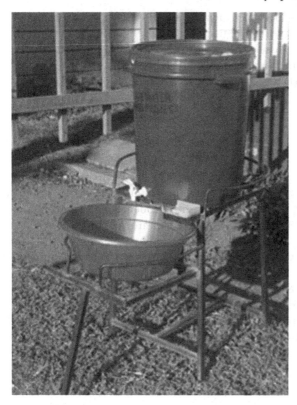

Figure 2.3 An example of a hand washing station with plastic bucket containing a tap, metal stand, basin for catching water and soap.
Source: CDC, 2015b. Retrieved from https://www.cdc.gov/safewater/stories.html.

unprotected source means putting contaminated water in the bucket for use which defeats the purpose of hand hygiene. In very poor settings, buying buckets enough for the whole school could be perceived as costly (see Figure 2.3).

Traditional approach vs current techniques of hand washing

There are several practices and techniques that people follow which have scientifically proven effective. Although some quarters of the society do not adhere, the proven procedures need to be followed in order to reduce the diarrhoea and respiratory infections among schoolchildren and the general population especially in developing countries. This would, in turn, help to reduce school absenteeism associated with infectious diseases. The health impact of hand hygiene within a school setting can be increased by using products and scientifically proven standardised procedures, either alone or in sequence, that maximise the log reduction of both bacteria and viruses on hands (Bloomfield, Aiello, Cookson, O'Boyle, & Larson, 2007). The hand washing procedures that will be discussed in this sub-section include: (1) seven steps, (2) five steps and (3) traditional way (Figure 2.4).

Seven-step technique

The World Health Organization (WHO) has long advocated for the use of a seven-step technique for hand washing. This has been incorporated in formal training in developed and developing countries as part of healthcare training (WHO, 2009). However, the incidence and prevalence of infections due to poor hand hygiene practices are still on the increase, especially in developing countries. Many studies have shown the low compliance of the seven-step technique among the general population and health workers globally (Kalata, Kamange, & Muula, 2013; Regidor, Vitalis, Lianah, & Mashood, 2014). While there are many factors that affect hand washing as presented in chapter two of this book, it is possible that the complexity of the seven-step procedure also contributes greatly to non-compliance, especially among young school-aged children (Lee & Lee., 2014 Lee, Leung, Tong, Chen, & Lee, 2015). This is more

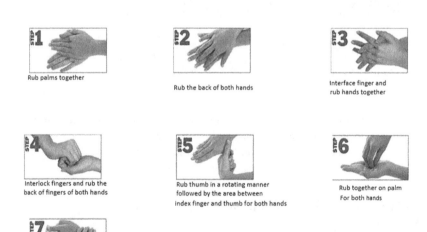

Figure 2.4 Seven steps of hand washing.
Source: https://www.pinterest.com/pin/71072500340388657/.

pronounced in young schoolchildren who learn better through simple and shorter instructions rather than complex procedures (Lee & Lee, 2014, Lee et al., 2015). Since children's cognitive and motor skills are not fully developed, it is very easy to get their long sleeves wet as they practise washing their hands and wrists using the seven-step hand washing technique (Lee et al., 2014, 2015). Wet sleeves create a conducive environment for microorganisms to live and multiply, thereafter being transferred through direct contact to the hands, then to the mouth or eyes, completing the epidemiological triad of the infectious disease transmission cycle (hand-to-mouth or hand-to-eye) (Figure 2.5).

Five-step technique

A simplified five-step hand washing technique was developed due to the need to reduce the number of steps in the WHO's seven-step hand

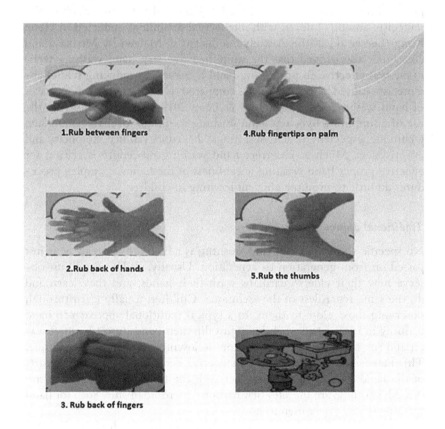

1.Rub between fingers

4.Rub fingertips on palm

2.Rub back of hands

5.Rub the thumbs

3. Rub back of fingers

Figure 2.5 Five-step technique of hand washing.
Source: Adapted from Lee et al. (2014).

washing technique, and which is validated in a pilot study by Lee and Lee (2014). The simplified five-step technique is simpler and easier to master/ memorise than the seven-step technique for children whose cognitive and motor abilities are not fully developed. Children at the elementary stage are still young and immature socially, physiologically, psychologically and intellectually. This makes them take longer time to follow instructions and master complicated procedures, being at the same time more vulnerable to infections. Therefore, the simplified five-step hand washing technique could be a better way of imparting hand washing skills than using the seven-step technique, which is longer and somehow more complex for schoolchildren in comparison.

While any validated and standardised hand washing is highly recommended, a simplified five-step hand washing technique has proven to be more effective in reducing the spread of infectious diseases compared to the WHO's seven-step hand washing technique (Lee et al., 2015). This is evident in a comparative efficacy study of a simplified hand washing programme for improvement in hand hygiene and reduction of school absenteeism among children with intellectual disability conducted in Hong Kong (Lee et al., 2015). A study conducted in Malawi by Mbakaya and colleagues also proved that the simplified five-step hand washing technique was effective in promoting hand hygiene and reducing school absenteeism caused by poor hygiene, compared to usual/traditional practices of hand washing (Mbakaya, Lee, & Lee,. 2019). Thus, this justifies the use of a simplified five-step hand washing technique over the seven-step technique, especially in school settings, due to its validity, simplicity and effectiveness. Much as a correct hand washing procedure is critical for effective proper hand washing (cleanliness of the hands), complex procedures do little to promote efficient learning in children.

Traditional approach

No specific technique for hand washing is advocated. Instead, it is just passed on from generation to generation. Usually, children will just observe how their elders/guardians wash their hands, and they learn and do the same regardless of the technique. Children usually learn through observing those close to them. In a typical traditional approach to hand washing in rural settings, children just dip their hands into a basin of water and rub them haphazardly without following any specified technique. This makes hand washing very ineffective because several critical parts of the hand such as at the back, between the fingers and finger tips are missed; yet these are the sites that harbour microorganisms. Soap for hand washing is also rarely used to none.

In other rural settings in developing countries, children can dip and wash their hands in the same basin after their elders. This potentially subjects them to contaminated water and consequently consuming germs/microorganisms. Some quarters though defend this practice as a way of stimulating children's immunity and make their immunity strong. However, this is a wrong approach of stimulating the body's immunity for children, because currently there are vaccines and sera. Equally the non-specific technique followed in this case is not effective as it does not target each and every part of the hand; instead, they just rub hands together. As such, microorganisms still remain on the hands even after the 'so-called' hand washing. A study conducted by Mbakaya et al. (2019) among others proved that this approach is not better than the five-step technique of hand washing.

The impact of hand hygiene in reducing infectious disease risks in school settings can be increased by convincing schoolchildren to apply hand hygiene procedures correctly, for example wash their hands using the correct procedure/technique and at the right time such as before eating, after visiting the toilet, after playing, before, during and after preparing food, after touching garbage, after touching a pet just to mention a few (see Appendix 2.1).

The fewer the steps, the better, as long as clean hands can be achieved after washing. Therefore, the simplified five-step technique of hand washing could be ideal for schoolchildren, not only in developing countries but developed countries too. However, the simplified five-step technique would benefit more schoolchildren in developing countries where resources are a challenge.

• Make a comparative difference in the steps among the different steps mentioned above.

Take-home message

It is recommended that school settings in developing nations advocate for scientifically proven standardised hand washing techniques in their curriculum. The step-by-step approach of washing hands ensures that each and every part of the hand surface is reached and cleaned thoroughly, thereby reducing the microorganisms on hands.

References

Biran, Adam. (2011). Enabling technologies for handwashing with soap: A case study on the tippy-tap in Uganda. In. Uganda: Water and Sanitation Program; 2011.

Bloomfield, S.F., Aiello, A.E., Cookson, B., O'Boyle, C., & Larson, E.L. (2007). The effectiveness of hand hygiene procedures in reducing the risk of infections in homes and community settings including handwashing and alcohol-based hand sanitizers. *Am. J. Infect. Control* **2007**, *35*, S27–S64.

CDC. (2015a). Diarrhoea: Common illness, global killer. Accessed from http://www.cdc.gov/healthywater/pdf/global/programmes/globaldiarrhea508c.pdf

CDC. (2015b). Hand washing: Clean hands save lives. Accessed from http://www.cdc.gov/handwashing/when-how-handwashing.html

Eshuchi, R. (2013). Promoting handwashing with soap behaviour in Kenyan schools: Learning from puppetry trials among primary school children in Kenya. *Doctoral Thesis.* Queensland University of Technology; 2013.

Golin, A.P., Choi, D., & Ghahary, A. (2020). Hand sanitizers: A review of ingredients, mechanisms of action, modes of delivery, and efficacy against coronaviruses. *Am. J. Infect. Control.* **2020**, Sep;*48*(9), 1062–1067. doi:10.1016/j.ajic.2020.06.182. Epub 2020 Jun 18. PMID: 32565272; PMCID: PMC7301780.

Kalata, N.L., Kamange, L., & Muula, A.S. (2013). Adherence to hand hygiene protocol by clinicians and medical students at Queen Elizabeth Central Hospital, Blantyre-Malawi. *Malawi Med. J.* **2013**, June;*25*(2), 50–52.

Lee, R.L.T., & Lee, P.H. (2014). To evaluate the effects of a simplified hand washing improvement program in schoolchildren with mild intellectual disability: A pilot study. *Res. Dev. Disbil.* **2014**, doi:10/1016/j.ridd.2014.07.016.

Lee, R.L.T., Leung, C., Tong, W.K., Chen, H., & Lee, P.H. (2015). Comparative efficacy of a simplified hand washing program for improvement in hand hygiene and reduction of school absenteeism among children with intellectual disability. *Am. J. Infect. Control* **2015**, doi:10.1016/j.ajic.2015.03.023.

Mbakaya, B.C., Lee, P.H., & Lee, R.L.T. (2019). Effect of a school-based hand hygiene program for Malawian children: A cluster randomized controlled trial. *Am. J. Infect. Control.* https://doi.org/10.1016/j.ajic.2019.06.009.

Morgan, P. (2020). The Mukombe - Zimbabwe's first "tippy tap": A description of its value and use. In. vol. 2020: Aquamor Pvt Ltd; 2013.

Pickering, A.J., Davis, J., Blum, A.G., Scalmanini, J., Oyier, B., Okoth, G., Breiman, R.F., & Ram P.K. (2013). Access to waterless hand sanitizer improves student hand hygiene behavior in primary schools in Nairobi, Kenya. *Am. J. Trop. Med. Hyg.* **2013**, *89*(3), 411–418.

Regidor, D., Vitalis, R.E., Lianah, S., & Mashood, A.S. (2014). A clinical audit on the compliance on hand washing laboratory in a private university in Peninsular Malaysia. *IJIRST* **2014**, *1*(7), 013, 63-71.

UNICEF. (2011). Water, sanitation and hygiene for school children in emergencies: A guidebook for teachers. In. UNICEF; 2011: 75.

UNICEF South Africa, Children's Radio Foundation. (June, 2020). Youth reporter handwashing survey. Smulders, J.R., & Simon Meyer, J. (2020). WASH/RCCE key informant rapid needs assessment. UNICEF South Africa.

WaterAid. (2012). Hygiene framework. In. London, UK: WaterAid; 2012.

WHO. (2009). A guide to the implementation of the WHO multimodal hand hygiene improvement strategy, 2009. Available online: http://www.who.int/gpsc/5may/Guide_to_Implementation.pdf (accessed on 19 December 2015).

3 Status of hand hygiene practices among schoolchildren in developing countries

Hand hygiene situation

There is overwhelming evidence that hand hygiene reduces the incidence of various infectious diseases such as diarrhoea and respiratory infection. However, hand hygiene practice in schools in developing countries remains scarce. School water and sanitation coverage is only 51% in less developed countries (UNICEF, 2015a). A report by UNICEF (2015a) revealed that only 21% of schools in developing countries have hand washing facilities. This situation persists in spite of the fundamental right of every child to a safe and healthy learning environment, including WASH services (UNICEF, 2013). Status below is the evidence-based synthesis of the hand hygiene situation in developing countries.

A published systematic review (Mbakaya, Lee, & Lee, 2017) on hand hygiene intervention strategies to reduce diarrhoea and respiratory infections among schoolchildren in developing countries found that hand washing interventions registered a reduction in respiratory conditions, gastrointestinal problems and school absenteeism in intervention groups compared to control groups, with reduces in incidence ranging from 53% to 73%. In a study conducted in Egypt, elementary schoolchildren in the intervention schools were asked to wash their hands twice a day, and health messages were delivered through entertainment activities. The results revealed that in the intervention group, overall absences caused by influenza-like illnesses decreased (reduced 40%, $p<0.0001$), as did those caused by diarrhoea (reduced 30%, $p<0.0001$), conjunctivitis (reduced 67%, $p<0.0001$) and laboratory-confirmed influenza (reduced 50%, $p<0.0001$). It was concluded that an intensive hand washing campaign was effective in reducing absenteeism caused by these illnesses (Talaat et al., 2011).

Saboori et al. (2013) conducted a study in Kenya to assess whether supplying soap to primary schools on a regular basis increased pupils' hand washing and decreased *Escherichia coli* hand contamination. Multiple rounds of structured observations of hand washing events after latrine use were conducted in 60 Kenyan schools, and hand rinse samples were collected once in a subset of schools. The proportion of pupils observed to practice hand washing with soap (HWWS) was significantly higher

DOI: 10.4324/b23319-3

in schools that received a soap provision intervention (32%) and schools that received soap and latrine cleaning materials (38%) compared with controls (3%). Girls and boys had similar hand washing rates. Their study concluded that removing barriers to soap procurement can significantly increase the availability of soap and improve hand washing among pupils (Saboori et al., 2013).

School-based hygiene and water treatment programmes increased student knowledge, improved hygiene and decreased absenteeism in a study conducted among 42 Kenyan schools (Patel et al., 2012). In the study, a curriculum on safe water and hand hygiene was instituted in the intervention schools, and water stations were installed. Patel and colleagues found that there was an improvement in proper hand washing techniques after the school programme was introduced. They also observed a decrease in the median percentage of students with acute respiratory illness among those exposed to the programme. Students in this school programme exhibited sustained improvement in hygiene knowledge and a reduced risk of respiratory infection after the intervention (Patel et al., 2012). The effectiveness of hand washing in the articles reviewed by Mbakaya et al. (2017) is well supported by the findings and report of Fewtrell and Colfod (2004) and UNICEF (2009), respectively. The two articles stated that hand washing is the single most cost-effective health intervention in preventing diarrhoea and respiratory infections. The hand washing intervention is relatively cheaper than other interventions in preventing diarrhoea and respiratory infections (UNICEF, 2009). In addition, the hand washing intervention, which is rated as the most cost-effective, is regarded as the most efficient in reducing the morbidity of diarrhoea, at 44% (UNICEF, 2009). This underscores that hand washing is the most important public health intervention.

Previous studies on hand washing done in several sub-Saharan countries indicated that only 17% of subjects washed their hands with soap after toilet use, and that 45% of them used water only (Curtis, Danquah, & Aunger, 2009). O'Loughlin (2006) found that in rural Ethiopia, hand washing facilities were available in only 21% of latrines, and no soap was found in any of these facilities. Less than 4% of the households had access to adequate hygiene facilities (O'Loughlin, 2006). In another study done by Vivas and colleagues among schoolchildren in Angolela, Ethiopia, 52% of students had adequate knowledge of proper hygiene (Vivas et al., 2010). While 99% of the students reported hand washing before eating, only 36.2% reported using soap (Vivas et al., 2010). A large number of students (76.7%) reported that washing hands after using the toilet was important. However, only 14.8% followed this practice in reality (Vivas et al., 2010). Sub-Saharan Africa has the lowest rates for coverage of improved sanitation. Migel and colleague measured the impact of a school water treatment and hand washing project on the incidence of clinic visits at school for diarrhoea in one private school in Kenya (Miguel & Kremer, 2004).

The study reported a 36% drop in local clinic visits for diarrhoea-related symptoms following the implementation of the intervention, as compared to the previous year. In the same country (Western Kenya), a study by O'Reilly et al., (2008) measured absenteeism in nine schools that had received a water treatment and hygiene programme. They found a reduction in absenteeism by 35%, compared with an increase by 5% in nine nearby control schools over the same time period.

Unlike in developed countries such as Hong Kong, where use of a validated seven- or five-step hand washing technique is enforced among schoolchildren and schools are moving towards standardisation across the board, such efforts to promote hand hygiene among primary school students are lacking in developing countries (Lee & Lee, 2014; Lee, Leung, Tong, Chen, & Lee, 2015; Mbakaya et al., 2017). Developing countries need to learn from developed countries and strive towards standardisation of validated hand washing procedures/techniques.

'Scarcity of hand hygiene resources': insights of a case study in Malawi

The current hygiene situation in Malawi is that the percentage of households with an improved toilet facility is at 8%. Studies conducted in rural areas in Malawi suggest that the real practice of HWWS at critical times is occurring between 3% and 18% of the time (Malawi Ministry of Health [MMoH], 2011). In addition, the percentages of the population that have hand washing facilities with soap and water at home are 7% and 2% in urban and rural Malawi, respectively (UNICEF, 2015). This poses a great threat to the public, and especially to schoolchildren, who are more vulnerable because of their immature immunity to defend themselves against infection and because of the school set-up, in which children spend most of their time, mix with other children and get exposed to many infections. These infections can, in turn, be transmitted to their family members and the general community, leading to serious outbreaks of various forms of infectious diseases, making the school set-up a major factor in infectious disease transmission, prevention and control.

The Malawi Demographic and Health Survey [MDHS] Education Data Survey (2002) indicates that 97% of students in Malawi were absent one or more times during the 2001 school academic year, and that 86% of them cited illness as a reason for absenteeism. Diarrhoea and respiratory infections are among the leading causes of illness affecting schoolchildren in developing countries, including Malawi (Black, Morris, & Bryce, 2013). These infectious diseases affect schoolchildren and the community in general, mainly because of poor hygiene practices.

Kalenga (2012) conducted a study in Blantyre, Malawi with the aim of assessing water, sanitation and hygiene (WASH) in primary schools. He found that all 11 schools involved in his study had a reliable source of water supplied by either a tap or a borehole, or both. He also found that water was accessible to schoolchildren and well positioned, within 5–20 metres of the classroom. However, only two schools had hand washing facilities, and none had hand washing soap. This underscores the magnitude of the hand hygiene challenges in Malawian schools. In addition, a study conducted in two state-run primary schools in Blantyre revealed that schoolchildren had a reasonable appreciation of hygiene issues. However, the high percentage of *E. coli* present on their hands (71%) revealed that this apparent knowledge was not put into practice (Grimason et al., 2014).

Therefore, integrating relevant simplified HHP into the school set-up could be one of the most effective interventions, simultaneously improving both the health and education of children (WHO, 1995), and in return promoting the adoption of hand hygiene practices among schoolchildren. However, the main challenge remains the available resources for hand hygiene.

The authors of this book conducted a focus group discussion as part of exploring experiences of school teachers, school principals and parents during the implementation of SBHHP (appreciating assets). These groups of participants expressed sentiments regarding how the SBHHP had improved their students' and children's health. All interviewed participants expressed their appreciation of the implementation of the SBHHP extended to the home by engaging the parents with the take-home package and briefing session from school nurses. Schoolchildren were excited about participating in the simplified five-step hand washing technique and said it was much easier to remember with a supportive environment (e.g. with the availability of health expertise, soap, water and hand washing papers) both at school and at home so that they would not get sick. Their parents also felt relieved that their children were healthier and took less sick leave days. The school personnel witnessed hand washing behavioural changes with better health outcomes after implementing the SBHHP (Mbakaya & Lee, 2019).

Take-home message

- Hand hygiene in school settings is poor in developing countries owing to lack of resources.
- With provision of resources, schoolchildren in developing countries are able to wash hands.
- Hand washing programmes that are successfully implemented in school settings in developing countries have produced significant positive results such as reduction in diarrhoea, respiratory infections, and school absenteeism.
- Edutainment approach can help improve the adoption of hand hygiene practices among schoolchildren.

• Inclusion of hand hygiene into the school curriculum so that it becomes part of the routine learning experience for schoolchildren. In addition, the school authorities should enforce the curriculum implementation, with emphasis on hand hygiene.

References

Black, R.E., Morris, S.S., Bryce J. (2013). Where and why are 10 million children dying every year? *Lancet* **2013**, *361*, 2226–2234.

Curtis, V.A., Danquah, L.O., & Aunger, R.V. (2009). Planned, motivated and habitual hygiene behaviour: An eleven-country review. *Health Educ. Res.* **2009**, *4*, 655–673. [PubMed: 19286894].

Fewtrell, L., & Colfod Jr., J.M. (2004). Water, sanitation and hygiene: Interventions and diarrhoea: A systematic review and meta-analysis. The International Bank for Reconstruction and Development/The World Bank 1818 H Street, NW, Washington, DC 20433.

Grimason, A.M., Masangwi, S.J., Morse, T.D., Jabu, G.C., Beattie, T.K., Taulo, S.E., & Lungu, K. (2014). Knowledge, awareness and practice of the importance of hand-washing amongst children attending state-run primary schools in rural Malawi. *Int. J. Environ. Health Res.* **2014**, *24*(1), 31–43, http://dx.doi.org/10.1080/09603123.2013.782601.

Kalenga, M.K.S. (2012). Assessment of water, sanitation and hygiene (WASH) in Malawi primary schools. University of Queensland, Australia. Retrieved from https://www.academia.edu/5044042/assessment_of_water_sanitation_and_hygiene_wash_in_malawi_primary_schools

Lee, R.L.T., & Lee, P.H. (2014). To evaluate the effects of a simplified hand washing improvement program in schoolchildren with mild intellectual disability: A pilot study. *Res. Dev. Disbil.* **2014**, doi:10/1016/j.ridd.2014.07.016.

Lee, R.L.T., Leung, C., Tong, W.K., Chen, H., & Lee, P.H. (2015). Comparative efficacy of a simplified hand washing program for improvement in hand hygiene and reduction of school absenteeism among children with intellectual disability. *Am. J. Infect. Control* **2015**, doi:10.1016/j.ajic.2015.03.023.

Malawi Demographic & Health Survey: Education Data for Decision Making. (2002). Available online: http://pdf.usaid.gov/pdf_docs/pnacr009.pdf (accessed on 15 February 2016).

Malawi Ministry of Health. (2011). National handwashingcampaign 2011–2012.

Mbakaya, B.C., & Lee, R.L.T. (2019). Experiences of implementing hand hygiene for Malawian schoolchildren: a qualitative study. *Int. Nurs. Rev* **2019**, Jul. doi:10.1111/inr.12538.

Mbakaya, B.C., Lee, P.H., & Lee, R.L.T. (2017). Hand hygiene intervention strategies to reduce diarrhoea and respiratory infections among children in developing countries: A systematic review. *Int. J. Environ. Res. Public Health* **2017**, *14*(4), 371, doi:10.3390/ijerph14040371.

Miguel, E., & Kremer, M. (2004). Worms: identifying impacts on education and health in the presence of treatment externalities. *Econometrica* **2004**, 159–217.

O'Loughlin, R. (2006). Follow-up of a low cost latrine promotion programme in one district of Amhara, Ethiopia: Characteristics of early adopters and non-adopters. *Trop. Med. Int. Health* **2006**, *11*, 1406–1415. [PubMed: 16930263].

O'Reilly, C.E., Freeman, M.C., Ravani, M., Migele, J., Mwaki, A., Ayalo, M., Ombeki, S., Hoekstra, R.M., Quick, R. (2008). The impact of a school-based safe water and hygiene programme on knowledge and practices of students and their parents: Nyanza Province, western Kenya, 2006. *Epidemiol Infect.* **2008** Jan;*136*(1):80-91. doi: 10.1017/S0950268807008060. Epub 2007 Feb 19. PMID: 17306051; PMCID: PMC2870759.

Patel, M.K., Harris, J.R., Juliao, P., Nygren, B., Were, V., Kola, S., & Quick, R. (2012). Impact of a hygiene curriculum and the installation of simple hand-washing and drinking water stations in rural Kenyan primary schools on student health and hygiene practices. *Am. J. Trop. Med. Hyg.* **2012**, *87*, 594–601.

Saboori, S.L.E.G., Moe, C.L., Freeman, M.C., Caruso, B.A., Akoko, D., & Rheingans, R.D. (2013). Impact of regular soap provision to primary schools on hand washing and *E. coli* hand contamination among pupils in Nyanza Province, Kenya: A cluster-randomised trial. *Am. J. Trop. Med. Hyg.* **2013**, *89*, 698–708.

Talaat, M., Afifi, S., Dueger, E., El-Ashry, N., Marfin, A., Kandeel, A., & El-Sayed, N. (2011). Effects of hand hygiene campaigns on incidence of laboratory-confirmed influenza and absenteeism in schoolchildren, Cairo, Egypt. *Emerg. Infect. Dis.* **2011**, *17*, 619–625.

UNICEF. (2015a). Advancing WASH in school monitoring. Retrieved from http://www.unicef.org/wash/schools/files/Advancing_WASH_in_Schools_Monitoring(1).pdf

UNICEF. (2015b). The human right to water and sanitation. Geneva: United Nations; 2015.

UNICEF. (2015c). Water and sanitation coverage. Retrieved from http://www.data.unicef.org/overview/hygiene.html

UNICEF Zambia. (2013). Retrieved from www.UNICEFAfrica/posts/441392 015933358

UNICEF. (2009). Soap, Toilets and Taps. Retrieved from http://www.unicef.org/wash/files/FINAL_Soap_Toilets_Taps.pdf

Vivas, A., Gelaye, B., Aboset, N., Kumie, A., Berhane, Y., Michelle, A., & Williams, M.A. (2010). Knowledge, attitudes, and practices (KAP) of hygiene among school children in Angolela, Ethiopia. *J. Prev. Med. Hyg.* **2010**, June;*51*(2), 73–79.

WHO. (1995). Global school health initiative; School and youth health. Retrieved from http://www.who.int/school_youth_health/gshi/en/on

4 Factors influencing hand hygiene practices among schoolchildren in developing countries

Factors influencing hand hygiene practices

More than 2.5 billion people worldwide lack access to improved sanitation facilities (UNICEF, 2009). In 2008, only 37% of schools in UNICEF priority countries were reported as having adequate sanitation coverage (UNICEF, 2009) (see Appendix 2). Globally, the rates of hand washing with soap at critical moments, such as before eating and after using the toilet, range from 0% to 34% (UNICEF, 2008).

Hand hygiene faces several challenges regarding its implementation. The challenges range from resources, knowledge (theoretical and practical knowledge) as well as psychosocial factors. While these problems exist globally, the situation is worse in developing countries. Unhygienic habits in which people are rooted are the biggest challenges in grown up population. However, among schoolchildren habits may not have been fully established; hence, there is room for behavioural change regarding hand hygiene. These schoolchildren will form a future adult generation who would have embraced good hand hygiene habits.

Promoting hand hygiene programmes remains a big challenge due to hindrances in transforming knowledge into behaviour change and ensuring accessibility of supplies and infrastructure (Zhang, Mosa, Hayward, & Mathews, 2013). Poor hygiene practices and insufficient sanitary conditions play greater role in the increased prevalence and incidence of communicable diseases in developing countries (Vivas et al., 2011). Appropriate and effective hand hygiene practice for schoolchildren is important in preventing infectious diseases such as diarrhoea and respiratory infections, which are the two most common causes of death among children in developing countries (Cairncross et al., 2010; Talaat et al., 2011). A study by Rao, Lopez and Hemed (2006) reported that diarrhoea is the second most common cause of death among school-aged children in sub-Saharan Africa.

The author of this book conducted a systematic review of literature (Mbakaya, Lee, & Lee, 2017) and identified factors, both barriers and enablers, that influence hand hygiene programmes among schoolchildren in developing countries. Below is a presentation of these challenges and factors as unveiled by a systematic literature review.

DOI: 10.4324/b23319-4

Resources

The hand hygiene resources needed for use by schoolchildren to keep their hand clean include

- Hand washing facilities
- Soap
- Clean water
- Hand rubs/sanitisers

According to a joint report by the World Health Organization (WHO) and United Nations International Children's Emergency Fund (UNICEF), sub-Saharan Africa has the highest number of people (319 million) without access to safe water in the world (WHO/UNICEF, 2015). Moreover, according to the same report, the number of people in sub-Saharan Africa without access to good sanitation has increased since 1990 and is now pegged at 695 million (WHO/UNICEF, 2015). In addition, places for hand washing where water and soap are available are in the wealthiest households (WHO/UNICEF, 2015).

Where water is available but limited, people prioritise for other domestic purposes other than hand hygiene. This is mainly fuelled by its scarcity or high cost of water resource. For example, literature indicates that in some primary schools, children are barred from washing their hand citing high water bills as a reason (Mbakaya & Lee, 2019). The author of this book witnessed this situation during the implementation of the hand hygiene programme in school settings around Mzuzu City in Malawi. I found that upon visiting some schools under the project, the taps were dry. Upon inquiry, it was found that the school authority had closed citing huge water bills. Schoolchildren were also barred from washing hand periodically in situations where the water was not closed.

Inadequate resources such as water, soap, hand rubs and hand hygiene facilities have been highlighted in studies by Oswald et al. (2008) and O'Loughlin (2006) and are some of the barriers to children's hand hygiene practice. Where water or water stations are not readily available, people may not consider hand washing a priority. Failure to prioritise washing hands, especially after visiting the toilet, before eating or feeding a child; before, during and after preparing food; and after changing and cleaning up a child who has used a toilet increases the chances of contracting or spreading diarrhoea and respiratory-related diseases (Centers for Disease Control [CDC], 2016; UNICEF, 2017).

Recently, efforts have been made to mount buckets with a tap in several places especially during the period of COVID-19. In the villages, several tippy-tap hand washing stations have been mounted although one can hardly see a soap on the tippy-tap due to poverty levels. This means that people in rural settings still wash hands without soap and without standardised techniques, despite the threat from COVID-19. Efforts and measures have to be put in place to ensure that the hand hygiene habit that the communities have initiated due to COVID-19 outbreak should be sustained. Recent studies are needed to consolidate and quantify the evidence on hand hygiene practices in the era of COVID-19. Is COVID-19 a game changer in efforts to promote hand hygiene behaviour among schoolchildren and the community at large?

Inadequate knowledge and attitude

Hand hygiene practice among schoolchildren is largely influenced by their knowledge and skill acquisition (Mbakaya, Lee & Lee, 2019). In Malawi, the findings from a cluster randomised controlled trial revealed that schools that did not receive SBHHP (intervention) had lower scores in knowledge, skill and practice/adoption (Mbakaya, Lee & Lee, 2019). While information about hand hygiene seems to have been disseminated to many schoolchildren in developing countries, the main challenge remains translating the knowledge acquired into practice.

Negative attitude towards hand hygiene is more likely to detour schoolchildren from practice. It is therefore important to influence positive attitude through imparting knowledge on why, when and how to practice hand hygiene. Training is likely to change the level of knowledge, which may positively influence the attitudes of schoolchildren towards hand hygiene, thereby promoting hand hygiene practice among schoolchildren. A study conducted in Kampala, Uganda found that participants who were taught hand washing were more likely to have better hand hygiene knowledge, attitude and practice (Nuwagaba et al., 2021). It is also argued that local beliefs (attitudes) are more important and that qualitative research needs to be conducted in order to have more effective messaging, to tailor into hand washing interventions. Just provision of soap is not enough (Phillips et al., 2015).

Psychosocial, contextual and technological factors

According to Hulland et al. (2013) and Dreibelbis, Freeman, Greene, Saboori, and Rheingans (2014), contextual, psychosocial and technological factors influence hand washing at five different aggregate levels of habitual, individual, interpersonal, community and societal (Hulland et al., 2013). A systematic review conducted by Mbakaya and colleagues in 2017 found that there was an interplay of all these three factors in the implementation of interventions in all studies under the review to influence hand washing behaviour, which were delivered at different levels. For example, the review found that under contextual factors, researchers made sure that they created a favourable environment for habit formation, with hand washing stations put in place and soap made available (Luby et al.,

2004, 2005). Under psychosocial factors, researchers trained participants in order to trigger self-efficacy, increase knowledge and induce a sense of perceived threat due to infections, and there was advocacy from the interventionist (Patel et al., 2012; Hulland et al., 2013; Pickering et al., 2013; Saboori et al., 2013; Zhang et al., 2013). The technology factors, which were highly applicable to all the studies reviewed, were evident through financing, the availability of hand washing facilities, accessibility, and demonstrations on hand washing procedure and how to use hand washing stations such as tippy-taps (Mbakaya et al., 2017). It was also found that the studies reviewed did not use many of the contextual and psychosocial factors as compared to the technological factors (Mbakaya et al., 2017). Therefore, psychosocial, contextual and technological factors need to be taken into consideration when planning and implementing hand hygiene programmes in school settings in developing countries.

A Water and Sanitation Program report (2009) found that many different reasons were given by students in Senegal for not washing their hands. Among the reasons were not wanting to listen to what adults have to say, laziness, rushing to go for a break, loss of playtime, the dirty and smelly toilets.

Lack of standardised hand washing techniques in the school communities

The systematic review by Mbakaya et al., 2017 also found that none of the studies that had used hand washing as an intervention had specified or described the hand washing technique used, that is, whether they had used the conventional seven-step hand washing technique based on the WHO. None of the studies stated that they had used the simplified five-step hand washing technique, which has been tested and proven effective in a study conducted in Hong Kong (Lee et al., 2014, 2015).

This is evident in developing countries even during this dangerous period of COVID-19, where hand washing is advocated without putting an emphasis on the hand washing technique. People are seen washing their hands the way they saw others or their parents wash hands without following a specific standardised procedure which would ensure that each and every part of the hand is cleaned/washed and consequently reduce the number of micro-organisms on the hand and reduce the risk of disease contraction and transmission. It is unlikely to achieve a good hand hygiene practice and more so a clean hand without following a scientifically proven standardised hand washing technique such as seven-step or five-step. A study conducted among Malawian schoolchildren found that those who mastered the skill of washing hands using the five-step technique were more likely to practice hand washing. They also reported that their hands were cleaner than before acquisition of the skill/technique (Mbakaya & Lee, 2019).

Effect of climate change

The water cycle is part of our everyday lives, but climate change may have dire consequences for everyday water access. Climate change impacts water access. Climate change can lead either to drought or flooding. Drought leads to water shortage, and where access to water is a challenge, people including schoolchildren may not prioritise hand hygiene. On the other hand, floods can lead to water contamination; hence schoolchildren may practice hand hygiene using already contaminated water and consequently making them prone to diarrhoea which can lead to school absenteeism and also death. Diarrhoea is one of the leading causes of school absenteeism and also death among school-aged children as well as under five children in under developing countries. Furthermore, floods can make water look dirty, which can physically not attract a schoolchild to use it because it is dirty and not appealing to children.

Enablers to implementing hand hygiene programmes

Enabling factors for proper hand washing, according to a study done in sub-Saharan Africa, were avoidance of disgust, such as dirt and smelly faeces; nurturing, such as teaching children to wash hands so as to avoid ill health; status, whereby clean people seem to be more accepted; association of cleanliness with better socioeconomic status; looking more attractive due to cleanliness; the comfort from feeling and smelling fresh hands; and fear of catching diseases (Scott, Curtis, Rabie, & Garbrah-Aidoo, 2007). In addition, students indicated that they washed their hands because they did not want to get ill and experience the double loss of classes and interactions with friends. Some students idealised that having clean hands would help them to keep their books clean and in return get better grades (Scott, Curtis, Rabie, & Garbrah-Aidoo, 2007). A combination of education, enhanced perception of the health threat, self-efficacy and perceived social pressure could improve hand hygiene compliance (Pittet, 2001). It is clear that interventions aimed to promote hand hygiene could save millions of lives (Curtis et al., 2009; Cairncross et al., 2010).

In a study done by Zhang et al. (2013), after a hand washing programme (HWP) intervention, schoolchildren reported a large increase in daily hand washing rates. The HWP comprised three main components of hand washing education, construction of tippy-tap hand washing stations and provision of soap (Zhang et al., 2013). In another study, it was found that the proportion of pupils observed practising hand washing with soap was significantly higher in schools that received training and hand washing supplies (Saboori et al., 2013).

The experience of the author of this book in implementing hand hygiene programmes in school settings in Malawi, sub-Saharan Africa established the following factors which helped to promote the adoption of hand hygiene practice among schoolchildren, in the city of Mzuzu.

'Being committed'

My experience showed that the commitment made by the school management team in integrating the components of the SBHHP into the school curriculum and daily routines for practising proper hand washing technique greatly helped to improve the hand hygiene practice among schoolchildren. The school management team for example provided time, materials and facilities to support the implementation of the SBHHP in schools. Teachers and parents also displayed a form of commitment in such a way that they continued to reinforce the components of the SBHHP to schoolchildren as integrated in the education programme during the implementation of the hand hygiene policy. As a result, schoolchildren acquired the necessary knowledge and hand washing technique to the extent that they expressed their willingness to share both proper hand washing technique and the practical knowledge they learned from school teachers and parents with their schoolmates and siblings at home (Mbakaya & Lee, 2019).

'Sharing responsibility'

During the implementation of the SBHHP, the responsibility to reinforce and monitor proper hand washing behaviours among schoolchildren was effectively shared between school teachers and parents. Integration of those materials into the daily routines and school guidelines for proper hand washing techniques reduced the spread of infectious diseases such as diarrhoea and respiratory diseases. The supportive environment in school and at home had facilitated these behaviour changes and improved hand washing practice. This led to positive behaviour change on hand hygiene practice among schoolchildren based on the collaborative effort between the school and home. In the long run, hand washing practice increased and was sustained (Mbakaya & Lee, 2019).

'Disseminating good practice'

We found that the school staff's and parents' positive attitude and commitment towards the SBHHP were very significant. They proposed that the hand hygiene campaign should be promoted as a partnership with health agencies and health centres in the community. Thus, the community at large would have the obligation to learn recommended hand hygiene practices and prevent outbreaks of infectious diseases such as diarrhoea and respiratory infections, thereby contributing towards reduction in children's absenteeism rates at school. During the interviews, parents stated that their children requested that hand washing resources such as soap and towels be made available at home. They emphasised to their parents that proper hand washing techniques could protect them and others from a range of diseases, and that it was everybody's role and responsibility in this campaign to promote proper hand hygiene in the community. The people in the community should be informed that there would be infectious disease outbreaks in the community if they did not wash their hands properly. Regular health education and health promotion activities should involve stakeholders and people in the community. In addition, the children wanted everyone in the home to do what they were taught at school, namely to follow the simplified five-step hand washing technique (Mbakaya & Lee, 2019).

Take-home message

* Resources such as water, soap, hand washing station, hand rubs/sanitiser
* Inadequate knowledge
* Psychosocial, contextual and technological factors
* Lack of standardised hand washing technique in community/school settings
* Enablers to implementing hand hygiene programmes

References

Cairncross, S., Hunt, C., Boisson, S., Bostoen, K., Curtis, V., Fung, I.C., & Schmidt, W.-P. (2010). Water, sanitation and hygiene for the prevention of diarrhea. *Int. J. Epidemiol.* **2010**, *39*, i193–i205.

CDC. (2016). Accessed from: https://www.cdc.gov/handwashing/when-how-handwashing.html

Curtis, V.A., Danquah, L.O., Aunger, R.V. (2009). Planned, motivated and habitual hygiene behaviour: an eleven-country review. *Health Educ Res* **2009**, *4*, 655-673. [PubMed: 19286894].

Dreibelbis, R., Freeman, M.C., Greene, L.E., Saboori, S., & Rheingans, R. (2014). The impact of school water, sanitation, and hygiene interventions on the health of younger siblings of pupils: A cluster-randomized trial in Kenya. *Am. J. Public Health* **2014**, *104*, e91–e97.

Hulland, K.R.S., Leontsini, E., Dreibelbis, R.; Unicomb, L., Afroz, A., Dutta, N.C., Nizame, F.L., Luby, S.P., Ram, P.K., & Winch, P.J. (2013). Designing a hand washing station for infrastructure-restricted communities in Bangladesh using the integrated behavioral model for water, sanitation and hygiene intervention (IBM-WASH). *BMC Public Health* **2013**, *13*, 877.

Lee, R.L.T., Leung, C., Tong, W.K., Chen, H., & Lee, P.H. (2015). Comparative efficacy of a simplified handwashing programme for improvement in hand hygiene and reduction of school absenteeism among children with intellectual disability. *American Journal of Infection Control.* doi: 10.1016/j.ajic.2015.03.023.

Lee, R.L.T., & Lee, P.H. (2014). To evaluate the effects of a simplified Hand washing improvement programme in schoolchildren with mild intellectual disability: A pilot study. *Research in Developmental Disabilities.* doi: 10/1016/j.ridd.2014.07.016.

Luby, S.P., Agboatwalla, M., Feikin, D.R., Painter, J., Billhimer, W., Altaf, A., & Hoekstra, R.M. (2005). Effect of hand washing on children's health: A randomised controlled trial. *The Lancet* **2005**, *366*, 225–233.

Luby, S.P., Agboatwalla, M., Painter, J., Altaf, A., Billhimer, W.L., & Hoekstra, R.M. (2004). Effect of intensive handwashing promotion on childhood diarrhea in high-risk communities in Pakistan: A randomized controlled trial. *JAMA* **2004**, *291*, 2547–2554.

Mbakaya, B.C., & Lee, R.L.T. (2019). Experiences of implementing hand hygiene for Malawian schoolchildren: A qualitative study. *Int. Nurs. Rev.* **2019**, *66*(4), 553–562, 10.1111/inr.v66.410.1111/inr.12538.

Mbakaya, B.C., Lee, P.H. & Lee, R.L.T. (2017). Hand hygiene intervention strategies to reduce diarrhoea and respiratory infections among children in developing countries: A systematic review. *Int. J. Environ. Res. Public Health* **2017**, *14*(4), 371, doi:10.3390/ijerph14040371.

Nuwagaba, J., Rutayisire, M., Balizzakiwa, T., Kisengula, I., Nagaddya, E.J., & Dave, D.A. (2021). The era of coronavirus: Knowledge, attitude, practices, and barriers to hand hygiene among Makerere university students and Katanga community residents. *Risk Manag. Healthc Policy* **2021**, *14*, 3349–3356, doi:10.2147/RMHP.S318482.

O'Loughlin, R. (2006). Follow-up of a low cost latrine promotion programme in one district of Amhara, Ethiopia: Characteristics of early adopters and non-adopters. *Trop. Med. Int. Health* **2006**, *11*, 1406–1415. [PubMed: 16930263].

Oswald, W.E., Hunter, G.C., Lescano, A.G., Cabrera, L., Leontsini, E.... & Pan, W.K. (2008). Direct observation of hygiene in a Peruvian shantytown: not enough handwashing and too little water. *Trop Med Int Health* **2008**, *13*, 1421-1428 [PubMed: 19055623].

Patel, M.K., Harris, J.R., Juliao, P., Nygren, B., Were, V., Kola, S., & Quick, R. (2012). Impact of a hygiene curriculum and the installation of simple handwashing and drinking water stations in rural Kenyan primary schools on student health and hygiene practices. *Am. J. Trop. Med. Hyg.* **2012**, *87*, 594–601.

Phillips, R.M., Vujcic, J., Boscoe, A. *et al.* (2015). Soap is not enough: Handwashing practices and knowledge in refugee camps, Maban County, South Sudan. *Confl. Health* **2015**, *9*, 39, https://doi.org/10.1186/s13031-015-0065-2.

Pickering, A.J., Davis, J., Blum, A.G., Scalmanini, J., Oyier, B., Okoth, G., & Ram, P.K. (2013). Access to waterless sanitizer improves student hand hygiene behaviour in primary schools in Nairobi Kenya. *Am. J. Trop. Med. Hyg.* **2013**, *89*, 411–418.

Pittet, D. (2001). Improving adherence to hand hygiene practice: A multidisciplinary approach. *Emerg. Infect. Dis.* **2001**, March–April; 7(2), 234–240.

Rao, C., Lopez, A.D., & Hemed, Y. (2006). Causes of death. In *Disease and Mortality in Sub-Saharan Africa*, 2nd ed.; Jamison, D.T., Feachem, R.G., Makgoba, M.W., Bos, E.R., Baingana, F.K., Hofman, K.J., Rogo, K.O., Eds; The International Bank for Reconstruction and Development/The World Bank: Washington, DC, USA, 2006; Chapter 5.

Saboori, S.L.E.G., Moe, C.L., Freeman, M.C., Caruso, B.A., Akoko, D., & Rheingans, R.D. (2013). Impact of regular soap provision to primary schools on hand washing and *E. coli* hand contamination among pupils in Nyanza Province, Kenya: A cluster-randomised trial. *Am. J. Trop. Med. Hyg.* **2013**, *89*, 698–708.

Scott, B., Curtis, V., Rabie, T. & Garbrah-Aidoo, N. (2007). Health in our hands but not in our heads: Understanding hygiene motivation in Ghana. *Health Policy Plan.* **2007** 22, 225-233. [PubMed: 17526639].

Talaat, M., Afifi, S., Dueger, E., El-Ashry, N., Marfin, A., Kandeel, A., El-Sayed, N. (2011). Effects of hand hygiene campaigns on incidence of laboratory-confirmed influenza and absenteeism in schoolchildren, Cairo, Egypt. *Emerg Infect Dis.* **2011** Apr;17(4), 619–625, doi: 10.3201/eid1704.101353.

UNICEF. (2008). Global handwashing day 15 October. Planner's Guide. Retrieved from www.unicef.org

UNICEF. (2009). Soap, toilets and taps. Retrieved from http://www.unicef.org/wash/files/FINAL_Soap_Toilets_Taps.pdf

UNICEF WASH Annual Report. (2008). Retrieved from https://reliefweb.int/sites/reliefweb.int/files/resources/B3CD1B186D897290C12575D20030FFE3-map.pdf

Vivas, A., Gelaye, B., Aboset, N., Kumie, A., Berhane, Y., Michelle, A., & Talaat, M., Afifi, S., Dueger, E., El-Ashry, N., Marfin, A., Kandeel, A., & El-Sayed, N. (2011). Effects of hand hygiene campaigns on incidence of laboratory-confirmed influenza and absenteeism in schoolchildren, Cairo, Egypt. *Emerg. Infect. Dis.* **2011**, 17, 619–625.

WHO & UNICEF. (2015). Water, sanitation and hygiene in health care facilities: Status in low and middle income countries and way forward. Geneva: WHO; 2015.

Zhang, C., Mosa, A.J., Hayward, A.S., & Mathews, S.A. (2013). Promoting clean hands among children in Uganda: A school-based intervention using "tippy-taps". *Public Health* **2013**, 127, 586–589.

5 Opportunities to embrace hand hygiene practices among schoolchildren

Opportunities

1 Children are willing to learn, especially if the system mixes learning and play. This motivates the children and they are more likely to pay attention and master the hand hygiene skills, including hand washing and apply appropriately. In the process, schoolchildren are more likely going to develop a good habit of hand hygiene since they are not yet grounded in bad habit and that they can easily develop new and better habits like that of hand hygiene at all recommended times such as before eating, after playing, after using the toilet.

2 Children learn from others by observation (visual learning). Therefore, if schools can be hand hygiene friendly, schoolchildren can easily learn from fellow students and teachers within the school setting. Encourage them to work in group, forming hand washing clubs, and wash hands in a group so that they learn and correct each other. Forming hand hygiene inter-class competition can also enhance the adoption of hand hygiene practices among schoolchildren in developing countries (Figures 5.1 and 5.2).

3 Children spend much of their time in school, approximately 6–8 hours or even more per day. As such, they are a common source of infection transmission to and from home and school. Therefore, they are more likely to contract the infection from others and also transmit infections to their fellow students and siblings at home. Therefore, targeting schoolchildren with effective intervention to promote hand hygiene would greatly reduce the disease transmission cycle. This can lead to many benefits not only to reduce infection but also to reduce school absenteeism which may come due to illness related to poor hand hygiene. In the long run, hand hygiene improves the school performance of children. School settings can be a good target for infectious disease prevention and control.

4 Most parents/guardians love their children and would definitely support their children's hand hygiene habit. Each and every parent would want to see his or her child grow healthy and do well in school. Hence, emphasising on the benefits of hand hygiene in

DOI: 10.4324/b23319-5

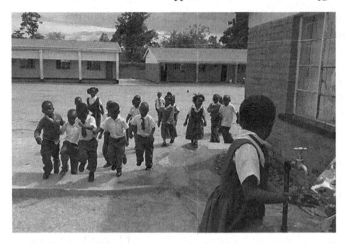

Figure 5.1 Schoolchildren mobilised to practice proper hand washing at a hand washing station outside their classroom in northern Malawi.
Source: Assoc. Prof. Mbakaya.

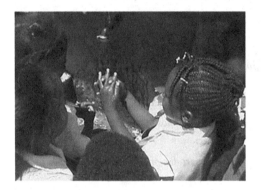

Figure 5.2 Schoolchildren practising proper hand washing in a group in northern Malawi.
Source: Assoc. Prof. Mbakaya.

disease prevention of deadly diseases such as diarrhoea can stimulate parent's commitment in supporting their children develop hand hygiene habit and also mobilising resources. As mentioned in Chapter 4, scarcity of resources is one of the hindrances to achieving hand hygiene practices in developing countries. Therefore, if the love parents have for their children be directed towards supporting their children's hand hygiene practices, they can easily join hands with schools in mobilising hand hygiene resources. In addition, the same parents will be able to help their child sustain hand hygiene practice even at home so that their child should not only practice at school (sustainability).

5   Children can be a channel for improving hand hygiene in their homes. Children can carry messages from school to their parents and siblings at home concerning hand hygiene. This can be in the form of knowledge and skills taught at school, but also leaflets and hand-outs with messages on hand hygiene. Children can teach their parents and siblings about what they have learnt at school.

6   Children can be advocates for good practice in homes. Children believe so much in what their teachers at school teach them or tell them to do. As such, children will always make sure that everyone at home follows what they were taught regarding hand hygiene. Children can even remind their parents and sibling to wash their hands if they have not done so prior to eating, after visiting the toilets, after playing. For example, during the implementation of school-based hand hygiene program in Mzuzu, Malawi by the author of this book, several excerpts were captured during the focus group discussion (FDG) showing children's advocacy for good hand hygiene practice in their home. Below are some of the quotes from the FDG:

If you wash like this (parent demonstration the old way) then you will hear from the child, mum mum you have not washed your hands (hihihi hehehehe- audience 6sec) you are supposed to do like this, all this area (parent demonstrating five step as taught by child)

P2W

Yes I will tell my neighbours and parents or brothers and sisters on how to wash hands so that they can also avoid those diseases

(C6bH)

when playing she calls friends and start demonstrating what she was taught at school (5-step)

P2H

And since that time he is always, each time he comes from the toilet goes to the sink, washes hands and he tells his brother, he has an elder brother, he tells him, have you washed your hands.

(P4R)

7   The Millennium Development Goals (MDGs) which have translated into Sustainable Development Goals (SDGs) have built considerable momentum and strengthened political commitment to child survival and development. The significant reduction in under-five mortality that has been achieved so far has saved millions of young lives over the past two decades. Much of this progress has been achieved by the adoption of basic health interventions in the context of general development, economic improvement, increased female education

and improved technology. This opportunity to advocate for and provide increased investment in pneumonia and diarrhoea prevention should not be missed (UNICEF & WHO, 2013). Along with this momentum, developing hand hygiene among schoolchildren can be promoted. An emphasis should be made that hand hygiene is the most cost-effective way to achieve this goal. This can be used to advocate for hand hygiene inclusion into different policies targeting schoolchildren in developing countries. This can be the opportunity to incorporate hand hygiene into school curriculum and allocate budget for hand hygiene resources in school settings.

8   The emergence of new COVID-19 pandemic should be an opportunity to accelerate efforts to promote hand hygiene which is currently touted by the WHO as the only best possible way of preventing the spread of COVID-19 besides other preventive measures such as social distancing. COVID-19 pandemic has heightened the importance of hand washing with soap (WHO, 2020).

The outbreak of COVID-19 pandemic in December 2019 has seen governments including those in the developing countries applying strict measures to contain the virus. Amongst the measures, hand washing with soap is a core intervention besides others. WHO has put much emphasis on hand washing as one of the most effective measures to contain the spread of COVID-19. With this, the community in the developing countries where resources are generally regarded as a major challenge to hand washing practice has seen different forms of effort towards achieving hand washing practice in trying to reduce the spread of the virus. Amongst the measures include using a plastic bucket with a tap and liquid soap at the entrance of shops, churches, schools and many other public places. In typical villages where they cannot afford to buy a plastic bucket, several tippy-taps have been mounted. The only challenge where tippy-taps are constructed is the lack of soap resources on the sites.

In addition, the technique people use for hand washing is still questionable as people do not adhere to a specific pattern/technique when washing their hands. Using the right techniques is very important to achieve a clean hand, but unfortunately, it remains a challenge.

Several committees have been commissioned to go round and monitor and reinforce this practice. People seem to comply with the orders put in place by governments. Developing countries need to take advantage of the measures put in place to reinforce and accelerate hand washing among the communities but with an emphasis on school settings. Furthermore, the governments should also reinforce a standardised hand washing technique such as a five-step hand washing technique or WHO's seven-step hand washing technique.

References

UNICEF & WHO. (2013). Ending preventable child deaths from pneumonia and diarrhoea by 2025 the integrated global action plan for pneumonia and diarrhoea (GAPPD). Accessed from https://apps.who.int/iris/bitstream/handle/10665/79200/9789241505239_eng.pdf?sequence=1

WHO. (2020). Covid-19 pandemic has heightened the importance of hand washing with soap. Accessed from https://www.afro.who.int/news/covid-19-pandemic-heightens-importance-handwashing-soap

6 Lessons derived from developed countries

Hand hygiene programmes in developed countries

It is well documented in previous studies that effective hand hygiene intervention strategies are well established in developed countries. For example, a report released by UNICEF (2015a,b) indicates that in developed countries, school water and sanitation coverage is at 89%. Allegranzi et al. (2013) conducted a study in five countries (Costa Rica, Italy, Mali, Pakistan and Saudi Arabia), in which they assessed the effects of WHO multimodal strategies for hand hygiene improvement. They found that compliance increased from 54.3% before the intervention to 68.5% after the intervention in high-income countries, and from 22.4% to 46.1% in low- and middle-income countries (Allegranzi et al., 2013). Hand hygiene compliance was independently associated with gross national income per head (Allegranzi et al., 2013). This is in agreement with the point discussed in Chapter 4, in which availability of resources is highlighted as an important driver to practising hand hygiene. It is easier for developed countries with high gross national income per head to procure resources for hand hygiene.

In a pilot study done in four United Kingdom primary schools, it was found that basic issues of personal hygiene were taught in the younger age groups, and that children of all age groups had good knowledge of hygiene practices (Schmidt, Wloch, Biran, Curtis, & Mangtani, 2009). Adequate and scientifically validated information on hand hygiene is crucial to teach the schoolchildren in order to improve their knowledge. In return, the knowledge gained will influence their attitude towards hand washing and start practising hand hygiene. In the process, schoolchildren would be developing hand hygiene habit. These schoolchildren would continue practising even after they grow up because they would have formed a habit. This would then be passed on to future generation. In this way, developing countries would have dealt with the chronic problem of hand hygiene non-compliance. There was a remarkable and sustainable behavioural and environmental change over a six-month period in a study done in Jerusalem among preschool children (Rosen et al., 2006). Their study found a three-fold increase in hand washing with soap among children in the

DOI: 10.4324/b23319-6

intervention group. This just emphasises that putting effort concerning hand hygiene on schoolchildren is rewarding in terms of results. School-children can easily learn and adopt the hand hygiene practice. Similar efforts and emphasis must be taken by government, policy makers and all relevant authorities in developing countries in order to increase the uptake of hand hygiene practice among schoolchildren in developing countries.

Lee and her colleagues considered different levels of hand washing-promoting practices that required multidimensional aspects such as insti-tutional support and capacity building in the implementation of the hand hygiene programme (HHP) in order to enhance the compliance of school-children in proper hand washing behaviours in special and ordinary school communities in Hong Kong (Lee, Leung, Tong, Chen, & Lee, 2015; Lee & Wang, 2016). Existing school committees such as Parent Teachers Association (PTA) should make deliberate effort as one of their agendas to mobilise resources for hand washing in schools. The PTA should play an advocacy role and engage different stakeholders in the school's catchment area and government to achieve lasting solutions to the challenges of the hand washing resources. School heads and directors should engage the health authorities in their area to help provide trainings to school teach-ers, parents/guardians and schoolchildren on hand hygiene. Ministries of education and health should work hand in hand to have the hand hygiene successfully implemented in schools. The two ministries should also agree towards standardising the validated hand washing procedure for use in their respective regions in developing countries. This approach is very crucial as it embraces multi-level approach to promoting hand hygiene among schoolchildren. Developing countries can heighten the adoption of hand hygiene practices through such practices and evidenced in developed countries.

A summary of approaches/lessons from developed countries worth emulating by developing countries to push for the adop-tion of hand hygiene practices in developing countries.

1 Having a school nurse responsible for each school or a number of schools would be a positive move towards achieving and scaling up hand hygiene compliance.
2 Health promoting schools to implement WHO concept.
3 Making resources available for hand washing (soap, water, sink, etc.).
4 School health/nurses associations to coordinate and enforce hand hy-giene practices across the country.
5 Standardisation of the hand washing technique. For example, seven steps mostly used in clinical setting. While five steps are recom-mended for community setting, including schoolchildren and it is proven effective. Simpler steps would help to promote compliance be-cause they are easier to learn, especially for young children in school environment.

6   How Hong Kong and other developed countries managed to contain SARS, H1N1, bird flu, etc.
7   School awards, trophies for the best school in promoting hand hygiene practices.

Developing countries need to take some of the lessons from developed countries and adopt or adapt some of the strategies listed above and other best practices that this book may not have included.

References

Allegranzi, B., Gayet-Ageron, A., Damani, N., Bengaly, L., McLaws, M.L., Moro, M.L., Memish, Z., Urroz, O., Richet, H., Storr, J., Donaldson, L., & Pittet, D. (2013). Global implementation of WHO's multimodal strategy for improvement of hand hygiene: A quasi-experimental study. *Lancet Infect. Dis.* **2013**, Oct;*13*(10), 843–851. doi:10.1016/S1473–3099(13)70163-4. Epub 2013 Aug 23. PMID: 23972825.

Lee, R.L.T., & Wang, J. (2016). Effectiveness of an adolescent health care training programme for enhancing paediatric nurses' competencies in central China. *J. Clin. Nurs.* *25*(21–22), 3300–3310.

Lee, R.L.T., Leung, C., Tong, W.K., Chen, H., & Lee, P.H. (2015). Comparative efficacy of a simplified hand washing program for improvement in hand hygiene and reduction of school absenteeism among children with intellectual disability. *Am. J. Infect. Control* **2015**, doi:10.1016/j.ajic.2015.03.023.

Rosen, L., Manor, O., Engelhard, D., Brody, D., Rosen, B., Peleg, H., Meir, M., & Zucker, D. (2006). Can a handwashing intervention make a difference? Results from a randomized controlled trial in Jerusalem preschools. *Prev. Med.* **2006**, *42*(1), January 2006, pp. 27–32. Retrieved from http://www.sciencedirect.com/science/article/pii/S0091743505001611

Schmidt, W.P., Wloch, C., Biran, A. *et al.* (2009). Formative research on the feasibility of hygiene interventions for influenza control in UK primary schools. *BMC Public Health* **2009**, 9, 390, https://doi.org/10.1186/1471-2458-9-390

UNICEF. (2015a). Advancing WASH in School Monitoring. Retrieved from http://www.unicef.org/wash/schools/files/Advancing_WASH_in_Schools_Monitoring(1).pdf

UNICEF. (2015b). Water and sanitation coverage. Retrieved from http://www.data.unicef.org/overview/hygiene.html

7 Recommended strategies to improve hand hygiene compliance among schoolchildren in developing countries

Multi-level intervention approach

Multi-level interventions are currently recommended for use in health care because client outcomes are a primary measure by which we assess healthcare delivery quality, and these outcomes are influenced by numerous other factors in the multi-level context of care (Edwards et al., 2012).

An intervention is multi-level if it addresses the individual client as well as at least two levels of contextual influence, such as organisations and providers, thereby targeting at least three different sources of influence (Edwards et al., 2012; Taplin et al., 2012). While multi-level interventions in health care are less robust, it is believed that they influence interdependent interaction, thereby producing desirable outcomes (Edwards et al., 2012; Taplin et al., 2012). A systematic review conducted by Mbakaya et al. (2017) attempted to look closely at the levels that were involved in the implementation of hand washing, and analysed them in order to determine whether multiple levels were used or not compared to the outcome of each study. Although the studies included in the review did not clearly state that they used multi-level interventions, the review found that almost all had implemented their interventions at three different levels, thereby qualifying as multi-level interventions. Five studies out of eight had managed to implement a hand washing intervention at four different levels by involving the individual participants, family and social support providers, and organisations. Two studies (Luby et al., 2004, 2005) were not very clear on how they involved the organisations/schools. However, they had managed to use three levels of intervention, as presented in Table 7.1.

In general, six studies found that hand washing was associated with statistically significant reductions in diarrhoea, respiratory infection and school absenteeism. Incidence of diarrhoea decreased by 53%–73% in the reviewed articles. Respiratory infection decreased by risk ratio (RR) of 0.77; CI = 0.62–0.95; EDM −2%; 90% CI = −3% to −1%. Reductions in school absenteeism due to diarrhoea and influenza-like infections were 33% (p < 0.0001) and 40% (p < 0.0001), respectively. These findings are consistent with literature showing that using a multi-level intervention and a combination of strategies improve efficiency and effectiveness, and hence

DOI: 10.4324/b23319-7

Table 7.1 Multi-level interventions and strategies used in the studies included in the review

Author (year) [study ID]	Multi-level				Strategies			Outcome of study
	Individual	Family and social support	Provider/ team	Organisation/ practice setting	Training/ education	Funding/ system change	Policy (reminder/ climate)	
Greene et al. (2012) [13]	√	√	√	√	√	√	√	Hygiene promotion had no impact on presence of any *E. coli* hand contamination (RR = 1.1; 95% CI = 0.7-1.8)
Luby et al. (2004) [15]	√	√	√	X	√	√	√	Lower incidence of diarrhoea was 57% (95% CI = -73% to -41%)
Luby et al. (2005) [14]	√	√	√	X	√	√	√	Lower incidence of diarrhoea was 53% (CI = -65% to -34%) and impetigo was 34% (CI = -52% to -16%)
Patel et al. (2012) [16]	√	√	√	√	√	√	X	Decrease in ARI (EDM = -2%; 90% CI = 0% to 0%)
Pickering et al. (2013) [17]	√	√	√	√	√	√	√	Hand sanitiser better than hand washing in reducing rhinorrhoea (RR = 0.77; CI = 0.62–0.95). Any loose stool (RR = 0.80; CI = 0.67–0.95). Soap better than sanitiser (RR = 0.77; CI = 0.62–0.95)
Saboori et al. (2013) [18]	√	√	√	√	√	√	√	Hand washing had non-significant effect on reduction of *E. Coli* contamination (OR = 0.43; CI = 0.15-1.23)
Talaat et al. (2011) [19]	√	√	√	√	√	√	X	Reductions in school absenteeism due to diarrhoea was 33% (p < 0.0001) and influenza-like infection was 40% (p < 0.0001)
Zhang et al. (2012) [20]	√	√	√	√	√	√	X	Absence of stomach pain (proxy measure of diarrhoea) (t = 10.8%; 95% CI = 0.92 – 1.68)

Source: Mbakaya et al., (2017). *Int. J. Environ. Res. Public Health* **2017**, *14*, 371.
Key: √ = Intervention or strategy was used in the study; X = Intervention or strategy was not used in the study; RR: relative risk; OR: odds ratio.

is likely to achieve the goals of the study or programme (Edwards et al., 2012; Taplin et al., 2012), in this case hand hygiene. Developing countries need to try implementing hand hygiene programmes in school settings using the multi-level approach in order to reduce non-compliance. When implementing hand hygiene in school settings in developing countries, they need to involve several stakeholders such as students themselves, their teachers, school authority, and parents. The author of this book implemented a cluster of randomised trials involving six schools in the northern city of Malawi using the multi-level approach. There were four levels of influence to students' hand hygiene practice, that is, students, teachers, school authority and parents. Practically, the components of a multi-level interventions approach for the planning and implementation of the school-based hand hygiene programme (SBHHP) in the study by Mbakaya and colleagues consisted the development of hand hygiene protocol, integration of hand hygiene care into school curriculum targeted at more than one contextual level, for example the children, families and community across the school systems level rather than one single level (Mbakaya et al., 2019). In their study, they used different strategies to plan and implement the multi-level interventions targeting different levels of system in the child's environment. They integrated teaching and learning materials of hand hygiene programme into the school curriculum targeting schoolchildren and their families, formulated hand hygiene protocol targeting school policy and community, created health promoting environment targeting children and their families, behaviour-change training on proper hand washing technique targeting individual child, peers and their families, development of stickers and posters of the simplified five-step hand washing technique targeting children and families, made available hand washing resources in school and home settings, and partnership with health policy makers, community leaders and parents (Mbakaya et al., 2019). This approach produced significant results. Student's knowledge, practice as well as acquisition of the five-step hand washing technique were significantly improved. There was adoption of the hand hygiene practice among schoolchildren.

Hand hygiene intervention strategies in line with WHO guidelines

Prior to writing this book, the author conducted a systematic review to ascertain and consolidate evidence regarding "hand hygiene intervention strategies to reduce diarrhoea and respiratory infections among schoolchildren in developing Countries" (Mbakaya et al., 2017). The systematic review identified and grouped the activities in the eight randomised controlled trial (RCT) studies/articles under review into major intervention strategies that were used to implement hand washing interventions. The major categories of the intervention strategies were in line with "A guide to the implementation of the WHO Multimodal Hand Hygiene Improvement

Strategy" (WHO, 2009). There were many activities observed in all the studies, which were used to implement the hand hygiene intervention. However, thematically, three main intervention strategies (training, policy and funding/resources) emerged from the reviewed articles.

Training

Training is a critical success factor and represents one of the cornerstones for improvement of hand hygiene practices (WHO, 2009). Nearly all eight studies under review had a training component. The only difference was the level at which it was implemented (multi-level). For example, different groups of people, such as teachers, nurses, parents and field workers, delivered the training to schoolchildren, and students were trained as trainers of trainers, together with their teachers. Children were told to wash their hands at recommended times, such as before and after eating, and after using the toilet. Schoolchildren require training on the importance of hand hygiene and the correct procedures for hand washing and hand rubbing. Clear education messages on hand washing help to induce behavioural and cultural change and ensure that competence is deep-rooted and maintained among all children in relation to hand washing hygiene. While all studies had training components, no single study that used hand washing in its intervention described the hand washing technique used in children's training, that is whether they had used the conventional seven-step hand washing technique based on the World Health Organization (WHO), or the simplified five-step hand washing technique, which has been tested and proven to be effective in a study performed in Hong Kong (Lee & Lee., 2014; Lee, Leung, Tong, Chen, & Lee, 2015). Training is an important strategy that can easily be integrated with all other essential strategy components (WHO, 2009). Governments in developing countries need to invest in training schoolchildren about hand hygiene in order to improve compliance and reduce diarrhoea and respiratory infections which are amongst the common cause of death in school age and also common reasons for school absenteeism. Training on hand hygiene with a standardised hand washing technique needs to be included in the school curriculum. Schools or local government assemblies need to employ nurses, or public health workers or environmentalist who should be monitoring the hand hygiene and the general school sanitation. Knowing very well that human resource is a challenge in developing countries, one nurse/public health worker can be employed for a cluster of schools and organise school cluster meetings to discuss issues affecting hygiene in schools.

Policy

Policy as an intervention strategy was visibly implemented in two ways: first by creating an institutional safety climate, and second by putting reminders in strategic places in the school environment. The institutional safety climate refers to creating an environment and perceptions that facilitate awareness-raising and consideration of hand washing improvement as a high priority at all levels, including active participation at both the institutional and individual levels, as well as awareness of individual and institutional capacity to change and improve self-efficacy (WHO, 2009). In most studies, empowerment was done by training teachers, children and parents to be trainers of trainers. Schoolchildren were also encouraged to make tippy-taps in a study done in Uganda (Zhang et al., 2013). They also encouraged the formation of health clubs, which were responsible for monitoring the use of hand hygiene resources. The involvement of schoolchildren encourages active participation and ownership of the intervention strategy or programme, thereby making it more likely to be sustained. Government in developing countries and all its stake holders are encouraged to put deliberate policies in place which can promote hand hygiene among schoolchildren.

Reminders in the school setting are key tools to prompt and remind children about the importance of hand washing and about the appropriate indications and procedures for performing it (WHO, 2009). All studies which were included in the systematic review conducted by Mbakaya and colleagues tried to deliver the content through a multimedia approach, which is encouraged when training children so that they are interested and thus motivated to get the most out of the lessons (Lee & Lee, 2014; Lee et al., 2015). Posters were put in visible locations close to the toilet, eating and hand washing places. Pamphlets were distributed to children and parents as reminders on when, why and how to wash hands.

Developing countries should make deliberate policies and by-laws which can reinforce hand hygiene behaviour formation among schoolchildren. For example, policy makers can reinforce that each and every school should have hand washing stations (plastic buckets with a tap, tippy-taps, etc.), hand washing posters around the school, a big billboard at the entrance of each school indicating that the school is hand washing friendly, every teacher should be trained on hand washing, children should get take-home hand washing materials to share with their parents at home for continuity of what they have learnt at school regarding hand hygiene. School heads/directors should encourage the formation of hand washing clubs in schools. There should be a cup/trophy where several schools should compete on best performer every year on hand hygiene and general sanitation. In a cluster randomised trial conducted by the author of this book, several reminders were used in trying to promote adoption of hand hygiene practices among schoolchildren. For example, posters were used and were put on the notice boards, near the toilet, near the hand washing station. We also had given them a take-home package to use together with their parents at home for support and sustainability of hand hygiene practice at home when they knock off from classes. Teachers were also reminding schoolchildren every morning before they started teaching, also when children were going for break. The content in all the reminders included when, why and how to wash hands. On the how to wash hands, schoolchildren were taught a specific hand washing technique to follow, which made sure that each and every part of the hand was washed and clean. These reminders and the approach used helped to yield positive and significant results on promoting adoption of hand hygiene practice among schoolchildren in northern Malawi city of Mzuzu.

Funding

Funding ensures that schools have the necessary infrastructure in place to allow students to perform hand washing (WHO, 2009). Compliance with hand washing among schoolchildren is only possible if schools ensure that infrastructure and a reliable and permanent supply of hand hygiene products are available at the right times and in the right locations (WHO, 2009). In a systematic review conducted by Mbakaya et al., (2017), almost all studies ensured that the experimental group was supplied with adequate resources such as alcohol-based hand rubs and soap and water throughout, so as to make hand hygiene as easy and convenient as possible. For example, in a study conducted in Pakistan (Luby et al., 2004), field workers supplied the families with soap as needed. Hand washing projects conducted in Kenya had funding from an international organisation to implement the Water Sanitation and Hygiene (WASH) project in their country, which helped to fund most of the resources. For example, they managed to install hand washing facilities and construct toilets (Patel et al., 2012; Saboori et al., 2013).

Most studies used more than one strategy to implement hand hygiene, which made it difficult to isolate and conclude the one type of strategy that was most effective. However, the commonly used and most prioritised combination of strategies was training, followed by funding and policy. Developing countries need to make efforts to mobilise funds to secure hand hygiene resources. Authorities in schools should also promote locally available resources which are relatively cheap, readily available and convenient. One such resource is a tippy-tap hand washing station. Encourage schoolchildren to construct tippy-taps in their homes so that they continue with the hand hygiene practice they would have learnt in school. Locally available resources and technologies can be made available with little effort.

They can also use plastic bucket with a tap as a hand washing station. However, school authority should make sure that the buckets are cleaned frequently and water replenished everyday to avoid contamination.

Where soap is a challenge, some communities have used white ash and it worked to keep the hand clean and reduce microorganisms on the hand. In worst scenarios, poor communities have ended up washing their hands with wet soil/mad (reference). But it should be emphasised here that these two options (white ash and wet soil/mad) need further research to test their effectiveness.

In efforts to mobilise resources for hand hygiene, there is need to initiate "school friendly companies" approach to adopt a school which they should periodically help with hand hygiene resources. This should be possible because companies are supposed to help with these resources as part of their social cooperate responsibility. Companies in return can advertise some of the products at the school premises such as adverts on the walls outside the school fence, or open bank accounts for schools if they are banking companies, etc. This can help schools that are struggling with resources to be supported and consequently make them available and promote hand hygiene practices among schoolchildren.

The other approach to resource mobilisation could be writing grant proposal application to UNICEF, WHO, and other local organisations implementing child health programs/projects, so that they can fund or provide resources for hand hygiene projects in school. Soap manufacturing companies and plastic bucket manufacturing companies can be some of the target companies that can be reached out to support the school hand hygiene initiatives with resources to use in school and promote the adoption of hand hygiene practices. Addressing hindrances that affect hand washing among schoolchildren can be vital in promoting health and reducing school absenteeism due to infectious diseases. There is overwhelming evidence that hand washing can reduce the amount of microorganisms on the hands, in turn reducing the incidence of diarrhoea, respiratory infection and school absenteeism (Luby et al., 2004, 2005; Patel et al., 2012; Zheng et al., 2012). This means that if correct hand washing interventions can be scaled up globally, especially in developing countries, the lives of many children could be saved and morbidity reduced.

The findings of a systematic review on the outcomes of HWP, done by Mbakaya et al. (2017), indicate that the availability of human, material and financial resources is an important factor in successful hand hygiene behaviour. In the same article (Mbakaya et al., 2017), it was found that all studies in which they provided resources ranging from water stations to soap, tippy-taps and waterless hand sanitiser plus education on hand hygiene positively impacted on the outcome measures of the hand hygiene behaviour. Compliance with hand washing among children and the community at large is only possible if infrastructure and a reliable and permanent supply of hand hygiene products are available at the right time and in the right location (WHO, 2009).

Health promoting school (HPS)

A health promoting school (HPS) framework is a multifaceted approach that supports health behaviours (WHO, 1996b). It is important that staff in health and education agreed to the frameworks and work collaboratively to support best health and education outcomes for children in schools.

Schools are unique settings to foster the younger generations' participation in furthering their own health and sustainability. The HPS's framework and supporting resources guide the school through a whole-school approach to promoting the health, well-being and engagement of its students, including hand hygiene practices. There are three areas of intervention that are interconnected in the HPS: (1) school curriculum, teaching and learning, (2) school ethos, environment and organisation, (3) school community partnership and services. These three key areas of intervention are summarised in Table 7.2. The three areas of intervention described below recognise different levels of influence on health, moving from the individual to the school environment to the wider community context, and emphasising the need to act on all three levels to successfully influence health (WHO, 1996a).

Below are practical examples on how the three areas of intervention of WHO's HPS framework were applied in the doctoral thesis conducted by Dr B.C. Mbakaya titled "Evaluating the efficacy of a school-based hand hygiene programme for children in Malawi, sub-Saharan Africa: A cluster randomised controlled trial" (2018).

A practical example on how school curriculum, teaching and learning could be implemented

In a doctoral thesis conducted by Dr B.C. Mbakaya, schoolchildren were taught about proper hand hygiene with an emphasis on using soap and clean water and following the five-step technique of hand washing. This was done once a week for six months, with teachers reminding students twice a day during break and lunch, and during the morning assembly, for

Table 7.2 WHO's health promoting school framework

Area of intervention	Description
School curriculum, teaching and learning	Health education topic are promoted through formal school curriculum
School ethos, environment and organisation	Health and well-being of students are promoted through the hidden or informal curriculum which encompasses values and attitude promoted within the school and physical environment and setting of the school
School community participation and services	School seek to engage with families, outside agency and wider community in recognition of the importance of these spheres of influence on children's health

Source: Assoc. Prof. Mbakaya.

a period of nine months. The education content covered the why, how and when to wash hands. This helped to increase students' self-confidence and self-efficacy. This was more likely incorporated into school routine and schoolchildren were taught on daily basis and reminded to wash their hand at critical times such as after visiting the toilet, before eating and after playing. The school heads/directors and teachers reinforced the hand hygiene programme and became part of the school activities.

A practical example on how school ethos, environment and organisation could be implemented

In a doctoral thesis conducted by Dr B.C. Mbakaya, this domain was achieved through promotion of health messages beyond the classroom in the wider school environment, for example via posters, information displays, and school assemblies, teachers were trained on the SBHHP. The researcher also used peer-lead activism among students. During the study, changes to the physical environment of the school were also implemented, for example the researcher provided hand washing soap to schools for the entire academic year, constructed water pipes, constructed hand washing sinks and paid water bills in some situations to facilitate hand washing.

A practical example on how school community partnership and services could be implemented

In a doctoral thesis conducted by Dr B.C. Mbakaya on this domain, the researcher reached out to parents through schoolchildren by giving them a take-home package that contained the same information that was given to students at school and displayed on posters. An information sheet was also given to parents, with detailed information to read and understand before consenting to their child's participation in the SBHHP. Parents were also involved in the focus group discussion to hear their views, opinions and suggestions regarding the SBHHP. Meeting with the representatives of the Independent School Association of Malawi (ISAMA) was also organised to discuss the SBHHP implementation.

Having implemented the project, the outcome was a success owing to the effective implementation of the strategies here in suggested and recommended. These proposed strategies have been used elsewhere and brought positive outcomes. WHO also recommends these strategies and stipulated in different reports (WHO, 1996a, 2009).

Communication, social mobilisation and advocacy for hand hygiene

Through communication, community/social mobilisation and advocacy to address health issues needed at the individual, community and system levels has proven to be a successful approach in different settings and programs. Below is a detailed explanation on how each of the stated strategies can be applied in order to promote hand hygiene in school settings in developing countries.

Communication

A process of sharing ideas for common understanding, seeks to change knowledge, attitude and practice.

Standardised hand hygiene training package should be provided to the general community, teachers and schoolchildren. Intensive trainings should be conducted to increase schoolchildren's hand hygiene knowledge, change their negative attitudes and improve hand hygiene practice.

Community mobilisation

- It is the use of community network (leadership and groups of people) to encourage community support and action
- Seeks to promote wider participation and ownership by community members
- Set committees in place to oversee the hand hygiene practices through checking hand washing facilities in home, schools and other public places.

Advocacy

This section seeks to raise political commitment, social will and resources for health needs. This includes providing needed resources, developing policies and laws as well as raising public awareness of health-related activities. Developing countries should be applauded for the efforts made to promote hand hygiene during the COVID-19 pandemic. The government made deliberate effort to make hand washing resources available, developed policies on hand hygiene and by-laws were made in local governments to ensure that everyone practices hand hygiene. This seems to have worked. Along with that, similar efforts can be made even after the COVID-19 pandemic. In other ways, developing countries should continue to reinforce the efforts so far made in providing necessary hand hygiene resources, policies development and laws regarding hand hygiene. This should strictly be applied in schools apart from the general population. Developing countries should make hand hygiene a priority and give it all the attention it deserves and not only during the outbreaks of infectious diseases such as diarrhoea and respiratory infection. Developing countries are already suffering from these infections and cause a lot of disease burden and death. In addition, these two types of infections caused school absenteeism among school-going children.

References

Edwards, H.M., Taplin, S.T., Chollette, V., Clauser, S.B., Das, I.P., Arnold, D., & Kaluzny, A.D. (2012). Summary of the multilevel interventions in health care conference. *J. Natl. Cancer. Inst. Monogr.* **2012**, doi:10.1093/jncimonographs/lgs018.Greene, L.E., Freeman, M.C., Akoko, D., Saboori, S., Moe, C., & Rheingans, R. (2012). Impact of School-Based Hygiene Promotion and Sanitation Intervention on Pupil Hand Contamination in Western Kenya: A Cluster Randomized Trial. *Am. J. Trop. Med. Hyg* **2012**, *87*(3), 2012, 385–393. doi:10.4269/ajtmh.2012.11-0633.

Lee, R.L.T., & Lee, P.H. (2014). To evaluate the effects of a simplified hand washing improvement program in schoolchildren with mild intellectual disability: A pilot study. *Res. Dev. Disbil.* **2014**, doi:10/1016/j.ridd.2014.07.016.

Lee, R.L.T., Leung, C., Tong, W.K., Chen, H., & Lee, P.H. (2015). Comparative efficacy of a simplified hand washing program for improvement in hand hygiene and reduction of school absenteeism among children with intellectual disability. *Am. J. Infect. Control* **2015**, doi:10.1016/j.ajic.2015.03.023.

Luby, S.P., Agboatwalla, M., Feikin, D.R., Painter, J., Billhimer, W., Altaf, A., Hoekstra, R.M. (2005). Effect of hand washing on children's health: A randomised controlled trial. *Lancet* **2005**, *366*, 225–233.

Luby, S.P., Agboatwalla, M., Painter, J., Altaf, A., Billhimer, W.L., & Hoekstra, R.M. (2004). Effect of intensive handwashing promotion on childhood diarrhea in high-risk communities in Pakistan: A randomized controlled trial. *JAMA* **2004**, *291*, 2547–2554.

Mbakaya, B.C., Lee, P.H., & Lee, R.L.T. (2019). Effect of a school-based hand hygiene program for Malawian children: A cluster randomized controlled trial. *Am. J. Infect. Control*, doi: 10.1016/j.ajic.2019.06.009.

Mbakaya, B.C., Lee, P.H. & Lee, R.L.T. (2017). Hand Hygiene Intervention Strategies to reduce diarrhoea and respiratory infections among children in developing countries: A systematic review. *Int. J. Environ. Res. Public Health* **2017**, *14*(4), 371. doi: 10.3390/ijerph14040371.

Patel, M.K., Harris, J.R., Juliao, P., Nygren, B., Were, V., Kola, S., & Quick, R. (2012). Impact of a hygiene curriculum and the installation of simple handwashing and drinking water stations in rural Kenyan primary schools on student health and hygiene practices. *Am. J. Trop. Med. Hyg.* **2012**, *87*, 594–601.

Pickering, A.J., Davis, J., Blum, A.G., Scalmanini, J., Oyier, B., Okoth, G., Breiman, R.F., & Ram, P.K. (2013). Access to waterless hand sanitizer improves student hand hygiene behaviour in primary schools in Nairobi, Kenya. *Am. J. Trop. Med. Hyg.* **2013**, *89*(3), 411–418. doi: 10.4269/qjtmh.13-0008.

Saboori, S.L.E.G., Moe, C.L., Freeman, M.C., Caruso, B.A., Akoko, D., & Rheingans, R.D. (2013) Impact of regular soap provision to primary schools on hand washing and *E. coli* hand contamination among pupils in Nyanza Province, Kenya: A cluster-randomised trial. *Am. J. Trop. Med. Hyg.* **2013**, *89*, 698–708.

Talaat, M., Afifi, S., Dueger, E., El-Ashry, N., Marfin, A., Kandeel, A., El-Sayed, N. (2011). Effects of Hand Hygiene Campaigns on Incidence of Laboratory-confirmed Influenza and Absenteeism in Schoolchildren, Cairo, Egypt. *Emerg Infect Dis.* **2011** Apr;17(4):619–625. doi: 10.3201/eid1704.101353.

Taplin, S.H., Price, R.A., Edwards, H.M., Foster, M.K., Breslau, E.S., Chollette, V., & Zapka, J. (2012). Understanding and influencing multilevel factors across the cancer care continuum. *J. Natl. Cancer Inst. Monogr.* **2012**, *44*, 2–10.

World Health Organization. (1996a). Improving school health programmes: barriers and strategies. *The School Health Working Group: The WHO Expert Committee on Comprehensive School Health Education and Promotion.* Geneva: World Health Organization.

WHO. (1996b). *Promoting Health Through Schools – The World Health Organization's Global School Health Initiative.* Geneva, 1996.

WHO. (2009). A Guide to the Implementation of the WHO Multimodal Hand Hygiene Improvement Strategy, 2009. Available online: http://www.who.int/gpsc/5may/Guide_to_Implementation.pdf (accessed on 19 December 2015).

Zhang, C., Mosa, A.J., Hayward, A.S., & Mathews, S.A. (2013). Promoting clean hands among children in Uganda: A school-based intervention using "tippy-taps". *Public Health* **2013**, *127*, 586–589.

8 Way forward

Leaders and policy makers in the developing countries need to make an extra and deliberate effort to improve hand hygiene practices among schoolchildren. To meet the global target by 2030, concerted effort needs to be pursed. Below is a list but not exhaustive on activities which need to be implemented with political will:

1   Continuous education campaign/awareness in order to influence knowledge, attitude and practice.
2   Accessibility to clean water
3   Availability of hand washing facilities
4   Availability of soap
5   Availability of hand sanitisers
6   Form country-wide/national school health association to comprise multi-disciplinary teams led by school health or community health specialist.
7   More scientifically sound, evidence-based studies need to be carried out in developing countries, especially in sub-Saharan Africa where very few studies have been done and it is therefore difficult to generalise the findings. Upcoming studies need to use more than one intervention strategies with a multi-level approach when addressing factors that affect hand hygiene, in order to scale up and improve hand hygiene practices among schoolchildren.
8   Use multi-disciplinary approach to mobilise resources for hand hygiene practices in school settings.

DOI: 10.4324/b23319-8

Appendix 1

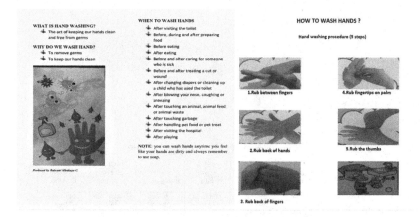

Figure A.1 An example of a simple leaflet to guide implementers in providing hand washing education in school settings in developing countries.

Source: Adapted from The Hong Kong Polytechnic University, School of Nursing.

Appendix 2

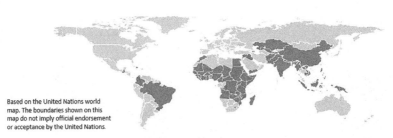

Based on the United Nations world map. The boundaries shown on this map do not imply official endorsement or acceptance by the United Nations.

WASH priority countries by region

CEE/CIS	EAPRO	ESARO	MENA	ROSA	TACRO	WCARO
Azerbaijan	Cambodia	Angola	Egypt	Afghanistan	Brazil	Benin
Kazakhstan	China	Burundi	Iraq	Bangladesh	Colombia	Burkina Faso
Tajikistan	Indonesia	Eritrea	Morocco	India	Guatemala	Cameroon
Uzbekistan	Lao P.D.R.	Ethiopia	Sudan	Nepal	Haiti	Chad
	Myanmar	Kenya	Syrian Arabic Rep.	Pakistan		Central African Rep.
	Papua New Guinea	Lesotho	Yemen			Cote d'Ivoire
	Philippines	Madagascar				D. R. Congo
	Viet Nam	Malawi				Ghana
		Mozambique				Guinea
		Rwanda				Guinea-Bissau
		Somalia				Liberia
		Tanzania				Mali
		Uganda				Mauritania
		Zambia				Niger
		Zimbabwe				Nigeria
						Senegal
						Sierra Leone
						Togo

Figure A.2 UNICEF WASH priority countries.

Source: *UNICEF WASH Annual Report 2008.*

Index

Note: **Bold** page numbers refer to tables and *italic* page numbers refer to figures.

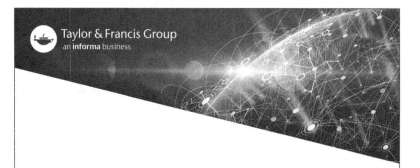

Printed in the United States
by Baker & Taylor Publisher Services